G000269751

In the Shadow of the

American Dream

In the Shadow of the American Dream

The Diaries of David Wojnarowicz

Edited and with an Introduction by Amy Scholder

Grove Press
New York

Copyright © 1999 The estate of David Wojnarowicz

Published simultaneously in Canada
Printed in the United States of America

FIRST PAPERBACK EDITION

Library of Congress Cataloging-in-Publication Data

Wojnarowicz, David.
    In the shadow of the American dream : the diaries of David
Wojnarowicz / edited and with an introduction by Amy Scholder.
        p.   cm.
    ISBN 0-8021-3671-0 (pbk.)
        1. Wojnarowicz, David—Diaries.   2. Authors, American—20th
century—Diaries.   3. AIDS (Disease)—Patients—United States—
Diaries.   4. Gay men—United States—Diaries.   5. Artists—United
States—Diaries.   I. Scholder, Amy.   II. Title
PS3573.04425Z47   1998
818'.5403—dc 21
[b]   98-25647
                                                                          CIP

DESIGN BY LAURA HAMMOND HOUGH

Grove Press
841 Broadway
New York, NY 10003

00 01 02 03 10 9 8 7 6 5 4 3 2 1

Editor's Note

Of the thirty-one diaries excerpted here, this selection represents perhaps ten or fifteen percent of all the writing. I have organized the journals as chapters, with dates and a title when there is one. I have made some notes within the text in brackets. Some of the entries I have introduced with notations in italics if contextualizing seems useful. I have tried to keep footnotes to a minimum to avoid interrupting the experience of reading the entries fluently. For the most part David Wojnarowicz used first names only of the cast of characters in his life. The last names appear here only when he made a point of using them. Drawings and photographs, expecially photo booth strips, postcards and letters, labels and ticket stubs, receipts and notes of things to do—all these items were filed within each diary. Near the end of his life, the author intended these totemic notebooks for publication.

Introduction

This book of diary writings by David Wojnarowicz comes from over thirty journals he kept from age seventeen, one summer in 1971, until another summer, in 1991, a year before he died. In the first diary (he saved, that is; there were probably earlier ones that weren't saved), David is on an Outward Bound expedition. He has high hopes for solitude and discoveries in nature but is then thwarted by severe conditions and physical hardship. He is unable to endure the diet and isolation, and he desperately wishes to get off the island, to return to the city from which he had wished to escape. Strangely, the end of his life reads similarly. His health deteriorates, and he feels more and more isolated and alone. With anguish he describes himself "disappearing." He realizes that, having gone through the experiences he has with AIDS and a culture that never deals honestly with death or dying, even if he were to survive, he would be filled with anger and hopelessness, anathemas to him. "I'm empty, other than of illness and dark thoughts. I want to die but I don't want to die. There's no answer right now" (August 1, 1991).

Anyone who turned the pages of these diaries would make different selections than I did, so it is important to introduce this set of writings, made from thousands of pages, as very much my own assemblage. I decided to follow a number of threads throughout David's journals that I believe are illustrative of the values he cherished, the struggles he endured, and the pleasures he sought.

The adolescent in the first diary is a typical boy fascinated with snakes and insects and what his body will do when put through an endurance test. But he is also a loner, not able to assimilate, a boy not fully aware of himself except for that queer feeling of not belonging and not particularly wanting to either. Expressing an interiority to the extent that he does in his diary is the first sign we have of David's literary talent for inscribing his condition on both a quotidian and a profound level. What he doesn't describe in this early journal, or in any of the subsequent chronicles that go into depth about who he is and what his dreams are, are the hardships of his childhood. In the biographical time line he provided for *Tongues of Flame*,* David gives a personal account of his youth: He is born in Red Bank, New Jersey, to a sailor from Detroit and a very young woman from Australia, in 1954. His parents get divorced two years later, leaving David and an older brother and sister in a sinister orphanage. His father visits occasionally, a year or two later kidnaps the children from the orphanage and brings them to Detroit, where they live with uncles and aunts in an unstable household until his father remarries a young woman from Scotland and moves his children back to New Jersey. His father is away sailing most of the time. When David is seven, his father forgets him and his brother and sister at a shopping center miles from home the day before Christmas. There is a blizzard, and his father is drunk.

David spends most of his time in the woods looking at animals. He starts hanging out with teenage boys in a local gang. An older boy tells David to play with his dick. A year later, another boy tells David to put his dick in his mouth. They do it to each other. By now he is eight years old, has taken up smoking, and his father has become more brutal, shooting off guns in the house, killing family pets.

In 1963, soon after Kennedy is assassinated, David and his brother and sister find their mother's name listed in a Manhattan phone book and secretly meet her in New York City for a few hours. She takes them to the Museum of Modern Art, and David wants to become an artist after that. His father finds out about the trip, and one day when he is drunk, he puts them on a bus to Port Authority, where their mother meets them. They live in Midtown next to a Howard Johnson's where later Angela Davis will be caught in a wig and dark sunglasses. David is approached several times

David Wojnarowicz: Tongues of Flame, the catalog for a major exhibition of his work at University Galleries, Illinois State University, Normal, Illinois, 1990.

by strange men before he finally begins hustling. Living in Hell's Kitchen, discovering his homosexuality, and being encouraged by his mother to paint and draw, David, at age twelve, shows signs of depression and considers suicide.

In 1968–69 he lives on the streets in New Jersey, Long Island, and New York City, sniffs glue, smokes pot and hash, attends Black Panther Party demonstrations, and meets a married lawyer in Times Square who takes him to his home in New Jersey when his family is vacationing elsewhere. This relationship helps David regain some self-worth, and after nearly starving for a year, he is taken care of. In high school David becomes acutely aware of the inequities in society. In 1970, he drops out of school, where he studied art, and lives mostly on the streets. He is drugged once, raped, and beaten while unconscious. He leaves New York City occasionally to escape his life, works as a farmer on the Canadian border, gets a job as a bookstore clerk (in a legitimate bookstore) in Times Square, falls in love with a woman, has a relationship with her for six months, realizes he is truly queer, and goes freight hopping across northern states to San Francisco, where he lives openly gay for the first time and realizes how calm and healthy he feels as a result. He also realizes that being queer is "a wedge that was slowly separating me from a sick society" (*Tongues of Flame,* p. 117).

From 1974 to 1978, David reads avidly, Genet and Burroughs in particular, and he takes several hitchhiking trips between coasts, interacting with the poverty population and growing more and more angry about the greed and disproportion of wealth and privilege in America. He begins writing street monologues based on the stories of people who live and work on the margins of society, and taking photographs with a camera a street buddy has stolen for him. He keeps a diary regularly, recording the things that happen to him and his feelings about them, letters he writes but doesn't always send, and art projects he plans to make.

In 1977 David goes to Paris, where his sister lives, and he plans to stay there. After a magical time in Paris and Normandy with a man who speaks little English, David decides to go back to New York City. In 1978 David's ideas about art making shift: he becomes interested in constructing with words, drawings, photographs, and objects an alternative version of history that disputes the "state-supported" form, which doesn't take into account how minorities survive. David's father commits suicide. In 1979 David begins working on a Super-8 film in the abandoned warehouses along the Hudson River, which is also where he spends much time exploring sexual possibilities, creating stencil murals, and gathering stories that he later documents in more monologues.

The 1980s were a cruel time for the poor in America, thanks to Reagan administration policies. Social structures that protected minority populations were dismantled, and any vestiges of humane public policy were abandoned. David becomes more and more invested in documenting these realities in his work—the images, words, and objects he creates have deep meaning to a thoroughly divested underclass, who have less and less access to cultural production and mass media.

Despite his brutal upbringing, and perhaps because of it, David had an invincible will to take control of his life and make of it what most deeply reflected his ideals. Hanging out with junkies and aspiring artists on the Lower East Side, David always resisted their lethargy and nihilism.

Working at Danceteria, taking heroin and speed, he never lost his drive to make work, to understand the world around him, and to improve his self-awareness. He had and wrote about countless sexual encounters, and almost always described these scenes as "lovemaking," as expressions of himself moving toward another, of gestures, however anonymous and arbitrary, with potential to change him forever.

Memory figures large in David's life: As a young adult, because of the images he has to overcome in order to heal from his past. As an artist, because his memory is the basis for connecting personal history and social conscience. And, once he becomes ill with AIDS-related symptoms, memory becomes his lifeline. At twenty-one, while hitchhiking, David reflects, "I saw a face in a passing car that looked like someone I once knew. It's like that when you move on to other places in your life—memories of faces fading like thin ice sheets in winter sidewalk puddles, they melt, become only a part of the water so you can't separate them ever again, but they do remain there" (July 25, 1976). Memory is also a path to thinking about mortality. As a teenager, he wrestles with these thoughts: "If I turned from twenty-three to eighty in the simple sway from window to bed what lives would remain in my heart, what answers to the questions of solitude and movement?" (September 19, 1977).

David was preoccupied with death and dying long before his peers began to succumb to the AIDS epidemic. But once he loses his friend, mentor, and onetime lover Peter Hujar, and receives his own diagnosis, his visions become overwhelmed by disappointment and rage. It is an intensely creative final period for him, and the diary entries are stricken and mournful:

> I'm afraid I'm losing touch with the faces of those I love. I'm
> losing touch with the current of timelessness. . . . I won't grow
> old and maybe I want to. Maybe nothing can save me. Maybe
> all my dreams as a kid and as a young guy have fallen down to
> their knees. Inside my head I wished for years that I could sepa-
> rate into ten different people to give each person I loved a part
> of myself forever and also have some left over to drift across
> landscapes and maybe even to go into death or areas that were
> deadly and have enough of me to survive the death of one or
> two of me—this was what I thought appropriate for all my
> desires and I never figured out how to rearrange it all and now
> I'm in danger of losing the only one of me that is around. I'm
> in danger of losing my life and what gesture can convey or stop
> this possibility? What gesture of hands or mind can stop my
> death? Nothing, and that saddens me. (no date, 1989)

In 1987, I was editing a selection of writings on AIDS for *City Lights Review* (I had been working as an editor there since 1984), and I invited David to contribute to this forum. I was familiar with his visual art and had not been aware of his writings until he sent me a piece called "AIDS and the Imagination." This work later became part of his book *Close to the Knives*. I was awed by the power of his writing, and in our correspondence we became friends. Not until after he designated me to edit his diaries and any other writings that could be collected posthumously, after he died and left his estate to his lover Tom Rauffenbart, and I moved to New York from San Francisco, sublet Tom's apartment, and read through all of David's journals, did I discover David's dream to be published by City Lights, and why he'd responded so openly and generously to my query years ago. That request for material on a subject few of us had been able to articulate: What is the impact of AIDS on the arts? The culture had been altered dramatically by 1987, most abruptly by the loss of great and potential talent, and in a subtle and pernicious way in which a youthful generation became enraged and grief-stricken, seemingly isolated from history and biological families and a dominant culture who for the most part felt exempt from this tragedy and blamed the victims for their own devastating fate.

It has been difficult for me to finalize this manuscript. As a work in progress, it has been a way for me to hold on to a set of feelings and a sense of reality that are perhaps no longer current, but relegating them to the past is like saying it's over, and it's not over. Thinking back on five or ten years ago, I realize how different my world was, knowing dozens of people suffering with AIDS-related symptoms, going to hospital wards and memorials, and considering estates of artists who left behind unfinished work. Most of the people I have known with HIV are dead now, and thankfully the few people in my life with AIDS who have survived this long can afford new treatments, and are responding positively to them. (No cure is around the corner, but what a difference it makes for people with symptoms suddenly to feel better for a sustained period of time.) My experience with AIDS now feels falsely part of my past, but I am more than haunted by a decade of loss. How to express the ways in which the images of young people dying in great pain have affected me and my generation? Nothing equips a young person for the horrors AIDS induced, through illness and prejudice and cultural neglect. In retrospect, the eighties and early nineties feel like a Poseidon Adventure some of us survived, and yet I know that many, many more people will lose their lives to AIDS-related diseases, and that my experience in urban America is altogether different from what is going on globally.

How do we in this culture responsibly reflect on and honor the lives lost? How do we prevent ourselves from collapsing so many memories into a totality that effaces the individuality of each person we loved and now miss? These are some of the final questions David engaged in his work, and his frustrations in the end were compounded by his inability to overcome what was taking away his life. Most of us are bewildered by the enormity of such experience, and inaction is often the result. But David continued to write and make art and confront his feelings as long as he could. When he was no longer able to work, his alienation deepened:

> I feel like it's happening to this person called David, but not to me. It's happening to this person who looks exactly like me, is as tall as me, and I can see through his eyes as if I am in his body, but it's still not me. So I go on and occasionally this person called David cries or makes plans for the possibility of death or departure or going to a doctor for checkups or dabbles in underground drugs in hopes for more time, and then eventually I get the body back and that David disappears for a while and I go about my daily business doing what I do, what I need or care to do. I sometimes feel bad for that David and can't believe he is dying. (no date, 1989)

David faced his own mortality with remarkable insight. In completely original terms, he invested his personal explorations and observations with fierce political analysis. In the work he produced, he shed light on facets of experience in America in the late twentieth century for an underclass who will forever be invigorated by his legacy.

Amy Scholder
September 1997

In the Shadow of the

American Dream

David's first journal, his record of an Outward Bound expedition, was written when he was seventeen years old. The diary is illustrated with maps and drawings of the terrain.

August–September 1971
Hurricane Island Outward Bound School
Grenfell Watch
P.O. Box 438
Vinalhaven, Maine 04863

Thursday, August 19, 1971

The first day we were coming over by ferry. It was foggy and the mist whipped at our faces. I was cold as hell. I started talking to my friend next to me whom I met at the airport. Soon he left with his friend and I sat behind a car to keep out of the cold. I began a conversation with a boy who was to be in my watch; his name was Tony. He is from Long Island. He lives there in the summer with his parents, but during college term he studies art in Sweden. Soon after, we reached Hurricane Island. Our watch officer's name was Charlie. We immediately went to our assigned tents and changed into running shorts. We ran once around the island and went to supper . . . a very small meal. I was hungry as hell afterwards. We went to sleep.

Friday, August 20, 1971

We got up and ran around the island. Very exhausting. I finished a cigarette I had and was going to smoke one last one before we signed a pledge to commit ourselves to do to our best ability the challenges and feats. And to stick by each other. Well I had the cigarette in my mouth and a lit match, about to light it. Then one person in my watch said that he feels we should all stick together before we sign the commitment. So in fewer words, I should not smoke my last cigarette. Well, I argued and everyone except Tony sided with George (the guy who started the whole mess). I said, Lordy, Lordy, I'm cured. And turned around all disgusted and walked away.

The kids then came up and apologized about it and said that they realized one last cigarette couldn't hurt. It was too late anyway since I broke up the cigarette. We went to sleep after supper and after signing the book.

Saturday, August 21, 1971

I learned the first steps in rock climbing. The man who teaches it hit me on the top of the head for doing a wrong signal at the wrong time. I was really pissed off. I am drawing the steps of preliminary rock climbing: Ombeli means I'm hooked up and ready for you to follow. Uprope means Pull up slack rope. The man situated on top of the hill pulls slack. When the slack is pulled up all the way, the man at the bottom shouts, That's me. The man at the top then says, Climb. The man at the bottom begins to climb and says, Climbing. The man at the top says, Okay, and pulls in the slack as the man ascends. If you kick off any rocks you can call, Below. If you feel yourself falling you call, Tension. The man at the top will immediately brace himself for the impact of the rope when you fall.

We ate lunch and got our swim trunks on and went for a swim in the granite quarry. We ate a lousy dinner of boiled ham and sweet potatoes. Ugh! I began to get tired. Sleep.

Sunday, August 22, 1971

We walked up to the freshwater pond and I caught a snake. A little garter snake. He started puking so I tossed him into the bushes. Imagine that, a sick snake.

We had to tie this rope around each of our waists and one by one crawl onto a little rope over the pond. We had to get to the other side. If one fell in we all would fall in. I was scared because my nice work boots were on. Thank Swami that we made it across and just in time for lunch. I ommmmmed in my mind all the way through the ordeal. After lunch we went on a real rock climb. I was first to go up since I had a dentist appointment. I made it up with very little trouble. I then left on the *M.V. Hurricane* to get to the dentist in Rockland. The *M.V. Hurricane* is a tugboat or a type

of ferry. I felt seasick but here was my chance to eat all I wanted. I had half
the pot of stew and ten oranges. The most I ever ate in my life!

I didn't get my tooth pulled. Back at H. Island, we began to get ready
for the trip tomorrow. We leave on a pulling boat and come back Saturday.
Nightfall came quickly. We had a big curse-out fight with another watch.
The stars were really bright.

Monday, August 23, 1971
Camp Island

I left early this morning. The swells were about 5 ft. high. I threw up so
many times. Finally I passed out. I woke up as we drifted into a nice quiet
cove. It was beautiful. I had a nice dinner of burnt macaroni, steamed mus-
sels, and carrots.

Tuesday, August 24, 1971

I slept badly and woke up with a cold. I ate breakfast. We boarded the pulling
boat and set sail for the next island. We learned about mainsails, mizzens,
square knots, Boling knots, etc. Soon I fell asleep. Today I did not get sick.
We sailed farther and farther. I was the bowman. We soon sailed into Bartlett
Cove. This is the Girls Island. Unfortunately there were no girls today because they were out on expeditions, like us. I slept soundly.

Wednesday, August 25, 1971

We sailed all day long and all night, we sailed in around 1:40 to Orono
Island. We cooked stew and woke up around 4:55 A.M. When I got up this
morning . . .

Thursday, August 26, 1971

I blew my nose and then I lifted a small rock to throw away the tissue. All of
a sudden there were two beautiful snakes curled up. One was a green snake
with white-green skin and milky white underbody. The other was a com-

mon ring-neck snake. Very small, with maroon underbelly. Must have been to the point of shedding. What a find. I let them go. My cold was worse. The sunrise was beautiful. We ran 6 miles afterwards. My legs were about to break. We soon left to sail again. Again I wasn't sick. We arrived very early at the most beautiful island I have ever seen. The name is Isle au Haut.

There were brine shrimp in the water and crabs running around in the seaweed. Deer were on the island. We found part of a skeleton of a deer. We had a good dinner of stew. (Good night.)

Friday, August 27, 1971

I woke up and walked around for a few minutes. It was very depressing out. The sky was very cloudy and dark. We got on the boat and I became very seasick. I ate some raisins and soon felt better. All of a sudden a report came over the radio about a hurricane which might hit New York and the New England area. We got scared. So we decided to get back to Hurricane Island.

We made it back and had a good dinner of two hamburgers, a bowl of soup, oyster crackers, and pears. I had a great sleep.

Saturday, August 28, 1971

We went rock climbing again and I learned rapelling. This is when you walk off a cliff backwards with ropes attached to you. If you let go with one hand you are going to fall and kill yourself. I remember having dreams of falling off cliffs as a little boy and the sensation was like this. I almost started crying.

The people who contribute to this island are here today. We are having a fantastic meal just to show them how good the camp is run. I am now going to sleep. I have been eating green apples so I have lots of gas. Ugh!!!

Sunday, August 29, 1971

I think that since I have quit smoking, my appetite has grown immensely. I eat and eat, then 15 minutes later I'm starving again. This morning we had like a junior Woodstock. Guitar and flute playing. Tonight I am watching a movie, *The Living Desert*. It is about all sorts of animals. We went on an ecology walk for preparation for our three-day solo, which will be in a couple of days. I think around Tuesday. They will take us on the *M.V. Hurricane* (ferryboat) and drop us off one by one on each uninhabited island. We have to live off the land for three days. This will be my chance to get some sleep and rest.

The movie was kind of funny but I was so tired that I slept through the last half of it. I am now in bed, I am very drowsy, so I will be signing off. Good night.

Monday, August 30, 1971

Every morning at 5:30 A.M. we get up, run around the island, and then take a jump into the cold, cold ocean. Brrrrrrr . . .

Well, this morning as we were running, three boys decided to show off their athletic skills and took off faster and soon disappeared. We have a rule, to stick together while doing everything. Some other boys and I have already hurt ourselves falling while running, so we had to take it slow. Well, we had to do five pull-ups. Those three guys who ran ahead had to come all the way back and do the five pull-ups. They started bitching about having to run slow because of the slower guys.

I was elected as first mate next to captain so I stood up and ordered them to quiet down as is expected of me. One guy, a very good karate pupil, told me to screw myself and to say shut up to his face. I had been fed up with everybody, so I walked up to him and said, Shut up. He did a karate flip on me, but I grabbed onto him before I fell, so I broke the fall.

We will be going on a ropes course which nobody has completed without falling at least once. I will try to do it without falling.

I just took a short walk into the woods. I found a small freshwater pond with a granite rock wall around it. Nearby was a little frail bird's nest. I picked it up.

I am feeling really depressed. I just caught another green snake on my way to the rope course. It was much smaller than the other one I had caught on Bartlett Island.

I just finished the first part of the ropes course. For some reason my kneecaps hurt so bad that I can't jump or do anything like that. I got into another argument with a stupid kid named George. I caught a frog in the quarry.

I am seriously thinking about leaving sooner than planned. I hate this situation. I have stuck it out to my fullest capacity. But there is only so much I can take from some people. The course isn't hard but the people are lousy.

I had a good lunch and am now ready to take over the watch from another crew. The emergency watch is when you serve the meals and stay up all night to make sure that any ships that crash in the dark can be rescued. You also do any job on the island that needs doing.

I helped scrape all the paint off the boat that was washed up on another island. I will be leaving in two days for my solo. Solo is when they take you to the island and let you stay there for three days. I will enjoy being alone and having to find and prepare my own food. I will write recipes for the meals I will have had. I get worried that the maniac might come and kill me in the dark while I am on the island. For some reason I am not afraid of monsters in the dark, but I am scared of maniacs and insane people waiting in the woods, in the dark. I get scared that they will grab me and kill me. I don't know why and I can't shake that feeling. I am very anxious to get back in the city, where the cold gray buildings are of some comfort and the lights make me feel safe.

I ate so much at dinner tonight that I am busting. I can't eat another drop. I am finished with my section of the watch and am now going to sleep. Good Night!

Tuesday, August 31, 1971

I did not have to run and dip this morning. Instead we set up the dishes and silverware and served breakfast. I am on duty again. (The time is now 8:39.) So far no calls have been made except some lady telling her husband's friend that her husband was sorry about not calling because his mother forgot to give him the message.

Breakfast was the usual oatmeal, 2 slices of bacon, 2 pieces of corn bread, and milk or coffee. I sneaked a peanut butter and jelly out of the kitchen. I am really hungry. Maybe it's all this exercise.

I am now waiting for my friend to get back from reading poetry at the morning meeting. Tomorrow I go on solo. Hmmm . . .

I just found out that I am sailing tonight and camping on an island until tomorrow, when I will be placed on an island for three days (solo). I am generally excited about what type of sleeping spot I will have. Where I will eat. What I will eat. And how the weather will be. Will I be able to start a fire, etc.

Well, I am now packed and am ready to sail as soon as everyone gets together. A boy in my watch caught a garter snake. It got away. I feel weird because I want to leave as soon as I get back from solo but I still haven't spoken to Rafe, the director. I think I will speak to him as soon as I get back. I will continue as soon as I eat dinner or else find out where I will be soloing (which island).

We just finished getting under way. One boy fell overboard. I will be writing a letter for Charlie to give to the director (Rafe) while I am away since I did not have a chance to speak to him before I left. I am going to ask him to telephone my mother and get her permission for me to come home. I hope she says yes (as I really know she will).

It is dark now and I have just set up my tent. I am damp and slightly cold but this night we had steak and baked potatoes and fruit salad to eat, sort of like a last meal. Happy that I am on solid land. I had a few more arguments with some kids in my watch so I will be glad to get on solo.

Wednesday, September 1, 1971

I am now up. Today I shall be put on an island by myself. The name is Babbitch Island. I am cooking breakfast for everyone else. It is now 5:10. I just finished breakfast and am cleaning up. I found out that I will be going to my island by powerboat. Thank Swami, because the pulling boats we use are so damned slow. Ugh!

Well, I am about to have hot cocoa in a pan, what a way to live. I finished getting checked to see if I or anyone else smuggled food with them. Well, I will soon be on the island.

Are you alone?

Are you alone? asked the man and his wife as I trudged past their trailer.

Are you alone? asked the gulls.

Are you alone? asked the ocean.

Are you alone? asked the frogs.

If a man is alone in this wide earth, then a neighbor is of no help.

I am on my island and have set up my tent. I have already eaten a lunch of stewed raspberries. It could have used some sugar, but I was quite contented with it. I am on my way to catch some clams and limpets for dinner. Dessert will be some glasswort (seashore plant—edible). I have found an incredible clam bed about halfway around the island from where I live. The clams are about five inches long. I found that it is easy to get to clams and limpets only when the sun is over behind the raspberry patch.

I will draw a map showing what I know of the island. I really enjoy watching the seals swimming about the cove. I was quite shocked to find out there were seals up in Maine. I thought they were in Alaska, etc. But they swim back and forth and occasionally will climb a rock and rest. This morning we saw ten of them on our way to the islands. I will now go and cook my clams, using a cup of sea water for the salt flavor. I am using a huge mussel shell as a spoon or small dish.

There is an abundant supply of rose hips, a plant that bears tomatolike fruit. It tastes like a mealy apple. The petals of the flowers on rose hip bushes are tasty also. Rose hips are the chief source of vitamin C. So I will eat a few every day.

I am now eating dinner. The sun is as high as ever. I am now doing a drawing of a limpet after being boiled.

I have finished dinner. I had raspberries for dessert. I don't enjoy eating these wild foods. I keep thinking of Blimpies, Cokes, ice cream, candy. Oh, how I wish I were home.

It is strange but for some reason I have changed and I know it. I have taken for granted many, many things. I will be happy to go into a food store and buy an apple or a cupcake. I will be more than happy to be walking on streets where people sell plastic flowers and pretzels and jewelry. Where the days are darker than the nights at times. To be able to come and go as I please. No island to restrict me.

Thursday, September 2, 1971

Well I am up and ready for a day's work. This morning I will not eat but will take a walk around my island to find more sources of food other than glasswort, rose hips, limpets, periwinkles, clams, and raspberries. I have found a plastic jug which might prove to be helpful. If I cut it in half it could be a bowl. I will try to think what other uses it could have.

Last night I was feeling pretty sick for some reason. Not my stomach, but my head. It was all cloudy. I went to sleep at approximately 6 o'clock.

The checkup men in the powerboat just came. They come once a day to see if your signal flag is up. If it isn't up and you don't wave to them then it means something is seriously wrong.

I must really be psychic because I was walking down to put up my signal flag when I saw a long board. I went over to it thinking there might be a snake under it. Well, just before I got to the board something moved on the grass. I thought it was a toad, so on a close look, I saw part of a snake gliding through the leaves. I caught another green snake. I was tempted to keep it but I let it go.

I just found a huge supply of glasswort past my clam bed. Glasswort is tender, juicy, and already salted with healthful sea salt. Continuing past another cove I found an excellent cattail supply. Cattails can be husked and boiled ten minutes to produce a delicious meaty substance. Cattails grow in freshwater marshes so I will see if I can find any freshwater things to eat.

I have ended up on the other side of the island. I have tried fishing, but there is no luck. I am getting dizzy from time to time from need of food. It is difficult to get used to some of the available sea plants, etc. I dropped my roll of fishing line and it fell a long ways and started to sink. I started pulling in the line as fast as I could which brought the line spool to the surface. I grabbed it. It was hell trying to wind up all that line but I managed it.

I think I will go for a swim later on when I get back.

I feel so sick I can hardly walk. The sun is too strong. I have a terrible headache.

I am about a quarter of a mile from my tent. Thank Swami.

I will cook my food that I have gathered and eat as soon as I get back. I am famished.

I have finished eating and I feel like throwing up. I can't wait to get back to Hurricane Island and to the meals they serve there. I feel like taking a nap which I think I will do.

Across from my cove is another island. I see a signal flag. One of my friends must be on it.

I just woke up and feel a bit better. I am not so hungry so I will fast until tomorrow. Then that will mean one more day and I will be back again. It is very strange when you don't use your voice for a period of time. You begin to realize how quiet things are and how beautiful nature is. I hear all kinds of birdcalls while I am writing this. At times I try to answer the call but some are too beautiful which makes it difficult.

I am going for a short walk to find some more curios. I have collected some already. It is fun to find something different from anything you have ever seen. It is low tide now so I can get closer to the water. I finished looking because my strength seems to be draining. I threw up already. I don't know what to do.

My curios are just the regular things I have been finding. I do not have any feeling or urge to draw in my sketch pad. I keep thinking of good wholesome food. I can't stomach all these foods out here. I am stomach-sick of clams, limpets, raspberries, and Christ knows what else. I am at this moment sick of every goddamn thing in this world. I wish I were home. I will try to leave right after solo.

I have been throwing up left and right. I ate some cattails and clams. That's when I started getting really sick. I will see if they will let me go back tomorrow morning. I can't eat any of this food. I need the normal food they serve at H.I.O.B.S. and at home. I am going crazy. I absolutely have to leave.

I was getting used to the course but I have had enough. I had enough a week ago but I stuck it out until solo thinking I would enjoy the rest. My stomach is killing me. I can hear the juices gurgling inside me. Today I made contact with the island across the way. After the boat left I heard shouting. It was Ricky, my friend. I could barely make out his words but apparently a boy named John in my watch was put on the other side of the island. He made his way to Ricky's camp and stayed there all night. Apparently he is very scared and homesick. He was going to leave about three days ago but Rafe the director talked him out of it.

Anyway I heard him blow his whistle so he is trying to make contact but I feel too sick to go all the way down to the beach and shout my lungs off. I'd probably end up puking. I think I will go to sleep in a few minutes.

I would rather wake up in the middle of nowhere than in any city on earth.

Friday, September 3, 1971

Last night I went to sleep just before the sun went down. I was not scared. I had quite a lot of trouble getting to sleep because I was getting cramps in my legs and stomach. Also I was extremely hungry. I had about one hour's sleep altogether.

Late last night my plastic tent was illuminated by light. I thought it was an unusually bright moon. About a half hour later the light was in the same position. I wanted to see if it was a full moon so I put on my glasses and poked part of my head through the opening. It was not the moon, but someone's flashlight. I was terrified. So I did only what I thought of, and that was to call and say, Who is that?

The light switched off and whoever it was walked down past my tent and onto the path leading to the cove. I am still very frightened from that. I poked my head back into the tent and remained barely breathing for about twenty minutes.

I vomited twice early this morning. I am writing this while waiting for the boat to come. I did not put up my blue flag because I want them to stay ashore so that they can take me away from this place.

I am still very frightened. Tried lighting a fire, but I used up the rest of my matches. I keep thinking I am hearing things. Like walking around in the woods. I am seated on a homemade bench by the sea. The waves are coming in faster and the birds are beginning to chirp. Thank Swami.

If they don't take me off this island this morning I will swim across to the next island where my friends are. I mean it.

I just finished packing all my things. I have had to. I am going to leave this morning. When I get to Hurricane Island I am going straight to Rafe and demand that he call my mother for permission to let me go home.

I can't wait to get back to New York City again. I keep thinking about the 8th Avenue Bakery, the candy stand in the drugstore, and Smilers food store sandwiches. I am driving myself crazy with the thought of good food. So far there are only signs of lobster boats. The Meka powerboat is not in sight. When it comes I am going to explain what happened last night and tell them that I can't stomach the sea plants and animals. I pray to Swami that they will take me back. I don't care what anyone thinks about me. I'm just sick and tired of all this. I want to be able to eat when I want and where I want. I want, I need time before school starts to adjust myself to the city. It will be bad to be depressed and then go to school at the same time.

My legs are feeling like lead weights are draped around them. I can barely walk. I keep thinking what I am going to say to the people in the boat or back at Hurricane Island. I keep thinking of the city. And all of the food stores. I also think how the children starving in India, Biafra, S.E. Asia, and the U.S. feel. Here I haven't eaten in two days and I feel this sick? Imagine what they feel.

I will be so happy when I am at the airport ready to board the plane. I JUST CAN'T WAIT. I keep hearing jets and planes passing by and it is nerve-racking waiting for the Meka powerboat. The sun is 1/8 across the sky.

The Meka boat appeared and went to my friend's island to check if everything was okay. He did not come here. If anything happens to me I am going to bring charges against the Island or H.I.O.B.S.! I think this is pretty sickening. Here I am getting cramps, starving, and throwing up, and the boat misses this island.

The sun is getting stronger. My head is getting cloudy.

Excuse me, but the Meka just came. They said for me to sit down and drink water every once in a while. They said that they were going to check the north islands and would be back this afternoon. If I thought I could stay until tomorrow morning, I could, or else if I didn't think I could take it, they would bring me back. I am definitely going back. I really couldn't take another night of staying awake and having cramps.

NO SIR, NOT ME!

I need some good normal food in my stomach. I'm not going to feel bad that I am going back early. I have to if I want to feel better. Some solo. Here I thought I was going to enjoy myself. What a laugh.

No sign of the Meka yet. I really do hope it comes back for me. All my stuff is on the beach and I am lying here writing to pass the time. I keep thinking about food and I am going absolutely crazy. You know that you can have food just about any time you want in the city. If you are starving, you can steal some. But, out here on an island there is no packaged food, only what you can find. And that makes you sick. If they don't return for me then tomorrow I am definitely going home after a meal on Hurricane Island.

I am feeling worse and the water I have been drinking feels sloshy in my stomach. The bees are buzzing and landing on me. The spiders are crawling around on me. Also the sand fleas and strange insects. I am waiting to see that boat zooming in to pick me up. I feel like crying but I don't have the strength to. I also feel like cursing out the world.

I don't know what is happening. I feel like I am about to burst inside. I want to scream and curse and yell and stomp and cry. I could never fall asleep tonight unless I had some good food to eat. Please dear God or Swami or Buddha or whoever is watching, let them come back and pick me up. I can't take another hour of this. Please.

Where are they????!!!!!!

THE MEKA JUST ARRIVED. They told me that in order for them to pick me up off the island when it isn't an extreme emergency they have to pick up a license, which would take about four hours. They gave me two slices of bread and a nectarine. I am eating slowly. I will go to sleep as soon as I am finished. They will pick us up tomorrow. Thank Swami!

I just ate another pail of raspberries. They make me nauseous but I have been drinking water and eating a piece of bread. That is so I will be full and then I can sleep. I have not eaten my nectarine. I am saving that until just before I go to sleep (which will be soon). I just saw a man and his two kids walking below on the beach. I suppose I could have said something but to me they represent freedom from this island and I can't have that freedom until tomorrow morning. So I don't enjoy looking at them much less speaking to them. I will continue until tomorrow morning. Good night.

I fell asleep and just woke up again. It is still daylight. It is an amazing thing how just a flutter of a bird's wing or a chirp can wake you instantly if nearby. I have forgotten the city sounds. I feel pretty good right now but occasionally think about tomorrow and a Hurricane Island meal. Also about the airport and its coffee shop and candy stand. Also the donuts and coffee before I board the plane. Yum! Yum! I wish tonight will go very quickly for I am going to get grumbles from my stomach.

It's funny but I can tell the kind of boat out here before it ever gets into view. While waiting for the Lurcher to appear today, I knew it was a lobster boat when I heard its motors. Well, I will soon try to go back to sleep. I hope I get to sleep. OOOOOMMMMMMM.

The sun is a bright orange ball sinking quickly. I still can't get to sleep. Maybe when it's dark the birds will shut up and I will fall to sleep. This light is going to be unbearable. I can feel it in my bones. I did not throw up the food they gave me. It just goes to show you that it is only this food that I am not used to that gets me sick. I am sleeping in a new spot overlooking the ocean. It is getting very foggy out. I can hardly see the other islands. The birds above me are still yakking away every once in a while. The fog is covering the sun but it is still light out. I am getting gas. The sound of the small waves breaking gets to be monotonous but I keep hoping I will soon get to sleep. When I lay down I feel wide awake. But when I sit up I feel sleepy. I am starting to get cold. I shall soon snuggle back into my sleeping bag.

Good night for good!

Saturday, September 4, 1971

Thank Swami, I finally got to sleep last night after about an hour of tossin' and turnin'. The mosquitoes are biting the hell out of me. It is still very early in the morning. I could not get to sleep so I started dreaming of eating licorice (black). It was very filling and I finally fell asleep with my stomach "full."

This morning is very foggy. I hope it clears up so I can see the ocean again. Damn those mosquitoes.

I just busted a rock that I found on the beach and inside are little crystals. I don't know what kind, but I imagine they are quartz crystals.

The sun is starting to come up. I hope it is going to be a beautiful day. The mosquitoes are lessening. But the bites are itching like hell. I have washed them off with alcohol, but it doesn't faze them. I think I have a long wait for those boats.

I am starting to get hunger pains again, but I can put up with them with the thought in mind of going back to Hurricane Island. I hope they have a meal waiting for us back there because I am not going to do any work without eating first. I am thinking about what is going to happen to people around home now that I've decided to come home early. Will Jerry

Baron ask why did I give up? Are they going to lose faith in me if I give up? I don't really care what they say or think because it is I who has made the decision, not them, to come home early.

I felt it was best for me to start the school year with a happy (not depressed) mind and on the same day as everyone else. That way there is no reason for me to mess up. Plus, I am really longing to see the city for the first time in my life. Amazing! Any other summer and I would hate to go home to those dirty streets. But I realize how much I have taken for granted. In fact how much everyone has taken for granted. I think everyone should go to a course like this. It makes them appreciate the freedom they had at home. There is an incredible amount of freedom in the city. Stores when you are hungry. Movies when you are bored. Bookstores when you feel like reading. Bars when you feel like drinking. I could go on for days writing about the things in the city that people take for granted. I just can't wait to get back to it all. I will enjoy every speck of dirt on the streets and buildings. I will be happy to see all the old bums again. The pimps, prostitutes, and whores. I will be extra happy to see the Broadway Game Room. I will be happy to see my mother and brother and sister and Johnny and James most of *all!*

The seagulls are fishing right now. They follow the lobster boats because when the lobstermen pull up their traps they throw away the crabs that have gotten inside, so the gulls dive for the crabs. AM I GOING CRAZY? There are what appear to be hummingbirds on this island! They zoom from flower to flower getting nectar. I have to ask about this.

Lobster boats in the distance . . .

I just thought about one of my friends who wanted to see a green snake so I decided to try and catch one for him. I realize that these uninhabited islands usually have many snakes roaming about fearlessly because no one is here to bother them.

Well, I started looking and pretty soon something flung itself into the taller grass nearby. (I imagine?)

It was a snake but it was too fast for me. I was pretty well pissed off for not being more alert and having seen it before it saw me. Soon I was walking on the other side of my little field and I said to myself, There's a nice quiet swimming area, and I walked over and what do you know? A little green snake was sliding out down the tiny pathway. I caught this one!

The Meka or the Lurch is not in sight or hearing distance. I'm getting sick.

The Meka picked me and two other friends up and left us on another island while they go pick up more kids. I feel more sick.

Well, we are on the pulling boat and waiting for twelve more people, then they are going to tow us in. It's a one-hour ride. But the sooner we get started the better I will feel.

My snake almost escaped. I don't blame him for trying. I realize how it feels to be locked up. He will soon be free.

One more group of people and we are on our way.

My snake got loose on the boat. But I caught him all the way up in the bow. That poor snake is in the hands of Cricked and some other asses who, thank Swami, are not in my watch. I hope he gets back to me alive without any broken ribs.

The man in the lobster boat is talking about homemade apple pie with a scoop of vanilla ice cream.

I met Dr. Spock today and his wife, Jane. He was tall and bald with a little fuzz around his ears. His wife had long brown hair. I was quite shocked speaking with them. I had tea and donuts.

I have had my evening meal and it is a strange feeling eating so much. I am glad to be back on the island where there are three meals a day. Good night!

Sunday, September 5, 1971

After a long run and cold dip I have just finished eating breakfast (delicious pancakes and hot maple syrup). Yum, it was very good. I am on my way to clean up the tents. I will soon speak to Pete Willauer about leaving soon. Everybody tells me that I am going to have a rough time talking to him. But he is only a human being and I feel I have made a decision so things should work out. They better because I have a dollar bet on it.

I have spent the whole afternoon speaking with Mr. Willauer. He is trying to get me to stay. But I swear after the incident at lunchtime, I am definitely leaving this island. Community togetherness, ha! I am debating whether to eat dinner with them or not. I am hungry but I don't know. I am feeling like dirt, which is what Willauer is trying to make me feel like, so I stay. But I am fighting it off because I know inside that I have made the right decision. I think I will go to dinner. I am slowly getting more and more depressed. Sometimes you would like to kill yourself. I'm still trying to figure out if I'm that desperate. Things don't seem to be going right at home between Mom and Steve. I don't know . . . It seems that just from the letters, I'm back where I started from already. I'll still be happy to leave this place. I am going to go straight to the candy stand at the airport and buy a Milky Way bar. Yum! I feel like crying but I won't give those bastards the satisfaction of seeing me cry.

I am going to wait until tomorrow, and if I don't hear word of when I will be leaving then I am going to split on a Meka or some boat. I swear.

I hate even thinking about those kids. Everyone probably thinks that I am more of a kid than they are. FUCK THEM!!! I have eaten and am more or less with the group. Good night.

Monday, September 6, 1971

We ran and dipped and didn't eat. Because of Chris and George, who did not feel like running. I am dying of hunger.

In his early twenties, David spent time hitchhiking and hopping freight cars from the East Coast through the Midwest, out to Northern California. The following is an excerpt from one of those hitchhiking trips.

July 15–August 17, 1976

July 25, 1976

11th day. Best day yet—not necessarily in terms of distance but in terms of great people.

We left the Milford Foote Hostel and hiked almost all the way up to 96. Stopped and chatted with a fruit-stand lady and corn farmer while eating plums. Got picked up by a young local hipster who drove us up to 96 in his car—Dylan blasting on the tinny radio. Showed us stoned color photos of himself and others (one of a girl bending over for something at a gas pump), some of him smoking dope—fuzzy color photos. Let us off and said he was tired of the town after twenty-three years there and was going to go to California too. Amazing how when you meet people in their daily life situations they immediately want to do what you're doing when you're on the road. It's a break from systematized daily life and it does look inviting but you have to do it not just fantasize.

We climbed up to 96 got a ride after a half hour with a local who "never normally picked up hitchhikers but saw our packs." Drove us down 23 as far as North Territorial Road. We got picked up pretty quickly by an elderly couple who were nice—quite funny talking as the woman lay with pure white hair and white skin bundled in sweater in front seat adjusting air conditioner. Her husband took us to his grandson's house in Ann Arbor where his grandson, a musician, drove us to the 94 West entrance ramp. We walked over to a K mart and had ham and cheese sandwiches on the Wrigleys Super Market Sidewalk with milk, Golden Fruit cookies, and we made squeeze oranges (that's where you cut a sugar-cube-size out of a good orange and squeeze the hell out of it for the juice—delicious). We soon got onto 94W and got a ride with a local

19

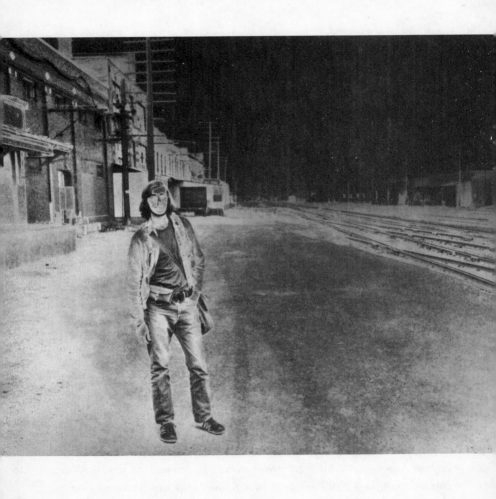

craftsman who worked in metal. He drove us a ways on 94 and then let us off.

We got picked up in a silver Mazda by a fellow named Stan Jones who sold stereo units and recording equipment in Indiana. He was up to visit a friend, Pink Floyd on the cassette recorder system. An incredible ride past sunburnt hills farms cars trucks zooming along and letting the mind drift. Back on North Territorial drop-off I saw a face in a passing car that looked like someone I once knew. It's like that when you move on to other places in your life—memories of faces fading like thin ice sheets in winter sidewalk puddles, they melt, become only a part of the water so you can't separate them ever again, but they do remain there.

Stan told us he was tired of working for others and that after next April he'll be home free. He and his friend in Ann Arbor (who's a real estate dealer) bought more than a hundred acres in Mexico. They made some investments together that paid off, bought a tractor, two Jaguars between them, a hydraulic pump for water-powered electricity (both were married). He said the land looked onto the mountains on whose base the land bordered. Said it was like a postcard of Colorado Rockies. They were going to build a huge home on the land with kilns for throwing pottery, an acre or two of garden vegetables, and an acre of third-generation pot seeds planted. The people they bought the pumps from would engineer the damming of the water for electricity. They were getting chickens and would use the manure for methane gas. He let us off near Lansing where we got a ride in an open-air Barracuda with a guy who had just gotten the car on the road with his cute red-haired girlfriend with freckled legs. Us three in front, John in back, we whipped off towards Kalamazoo, wind whipping our hair around.

Left off at Kalamazoo exit while they went on. A Kalamazoo county policeman pulled up just as we were walking to get off the interstate onto the exit ramp. Checked our ID. A young cop who watched too many TV police dramas, he said to us, You know, gentlemen, that it's illegal to hitch-hike on interstates. You could get fined (lifting mirror glasses from his nose) and you could even get thrown into jail, but I'm not that kind of guy. He told us to hop in the car and he would give us a lift to the exit ramp where we could legally hitchhike. We got in the backseat cage and he drove us the quarter mile up to the ramp, spoke into his radio, turned, and said, Well this has got to be a quick drop-off 'cause I have to get back. We tried to get out of the car but the police break the locks and handles off backseats of police cars so the suspects don't have a chance to run off. He had to get out and open the door for us. I was tempted to mock a royal accent: Thank you, Charles, but refrained.

July 31, 1976
17th day. Left YMCA St. Paul Hostel and headed for grocery store to buy provisions for freight hop to West Coast. Bought a bag of:

    12 rye pumpernickel rolls (small)
    1 can tuna fish
    1 box raisins
    1 can mixed nuts
    1 small bag peanuts
    1 small bag sunflower seeds
    1 gallon distilled water
    2 small cans peaches
    3 cheese cracker packages

Went and got a haircut at a slightly redneck place. The guy said (when I got up), Oh you're the one getting a haircut . . . ha ha . . . that's a surprise. Usually the guy who really needs the haircut doesn't get one and the guy with short hair does . . . ha ha . . . really that's happened before.

He gave me a classic short haircut while joking about the trials and tribulations of hitchhiking: You ever hear about the minister who picked up three girls who were hitchhiking and they held a knife to his throat and raped him? First he said, Sorry but I can't, but when they held a knife to him he did it. It was written up in all the papers around here. You never heard about it?

He charged four bucks for the cut. Also asked about hitching. How easy it was to hitch etc. I told him the best was as a pair—a girl and a guy, second best a guy, and that two guys represent hostility psychologically to motorists. His reply was, Well I guess one of you will have to start wearing a dress . . . ha ha.

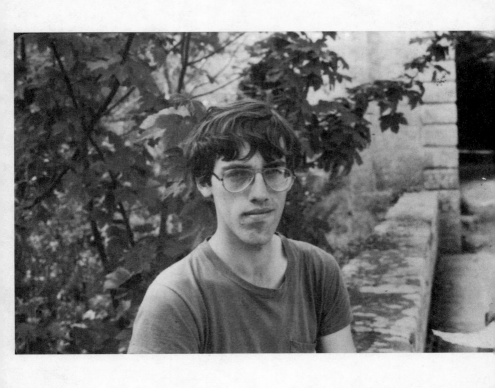

David lived in Brooklyn Heights in his early twenties and was hanging out with writers and artists, taking drugs, and going to downtown Manhattan nightclubs and gay bars. He started to take himself seriously as a writer at this time, and began collecting material for stories he called monologues.

July 26–September 4, 1977
Brooklyn Heights, New York
Human Head

July 26, 1977

Woke up early with a phone call from Herbert Huncke. He was calling to ask me to please meet him at the courthouse on 100 Center Street. He had been busted on 14th Street around 3rd Avenue a couple of weeks ago. The neighborhood is all broken bottles, yellowed milk-colored glass marquees, and coffee shops which are hangouts for the night crowds—those that gather slowly in the daytime moving from doorways of pawn shops to used magazine stores to tobacco stores to dusty apartments all heat-roached and sticky with summer weather. At night the whores come out along with pimps and everyone struts in high-heeled regalia under the glitter of a half-dead moon and fluorescent lights and lamp poles. Small kids with their trusty collarless dogs dash through it all. Avenues of pushers and between 3rd and 2nd Avenues—it's hot like wall-to-wall body tension, like people waiting for a connection somewhere in that wall of sound and flash. The cops had been after one pusher for a while and were watching him through the window of a closed-down shop. Huncke bought four Valiums and felt a hand on his shoulder just after he dropped them into a little brown paper bag. He dropped the bag to his feet and said, Wha . . . What's going on here?

Two cops said, Okay, where's that stuff you bought? I saw ya put it in the bag. Oh . . . here it is. Stooped down and picked the bag off the street. Huncke said, That's not mine, I don't know what you're talking about. The cop said, Now ya wanna make it rough on yourself or what?

By this time the other cop was relieving the pusher of bottle after bottle of pills, all colors and effects. They were booked and the cop said to Huncke that they didn't want to prosecute him just the pusher.

Met Huncke at the courthouse around 9:35 A.M. wandering down the hallway towards the room AP3, where his case was gonna be. We smoked cigarettes and hung around inside the courtroom all day long with a procession of cases in front of the judge. The judge was "lenient" as compared to most judges, but sentences were reeling out right and left along with fines. One girl who lifted a wallet stood holding her rosy black arms around her slim sides and traded back and forth with the legal aid lawyer with the sentence. She was caught up in it with no chance. Sixty days minimum. She didn't want it so they had her sit in a chair to the side to think about it while more cases were heard. She sat down and looked over the courtroom with the saddest eyes I've ever seen. I only saw a look like that on cattle before shot between the eyes with a hammer upstate on a slaughter.

A lot of people paid their fines and took their sentences without any arguments. The prosecutor district attorney hung out leafing through volumes of papers inside folders recommending this or that for the defendants. He was blond and very handsome but looked like he was straight out of the colonial-style suburbs of Long Island where lawn sprinklers whizz—whizz all day around vast columnar houses and little kids run through shady quiet streets oblivious to anything even faintly resembling the dome of New York City.

Huncke's legs jumped up and down and his fingers twisted around in half-knots from tension. Periodically he rushed downstairs to the bathroom or out in the hall with me for a cigarette. His legal aid lawyer didn't show up once all day and during lunch recess Huncke frantically called his office and asked other legal aid lawyers to give this guy a message that he was waiting for the man.

The tension was so unbelievable I wanted to put my fist through a wall. Poor Huncke and I were dancing in our seats, twisting right and left with apprehension.

The lawyer showed around 4 o'clock and Huncke showed him the two letters—one from a methadone clinic he was in at this time, and the other from a professor of English in New Jersey. Both had good effect on the judge and the district attorney who let Huncke plead disorderly conduct and let him off. I rubbed his back and hugged him in the hallway and we crash-stumbled around trying to get out of the fucking building as soon

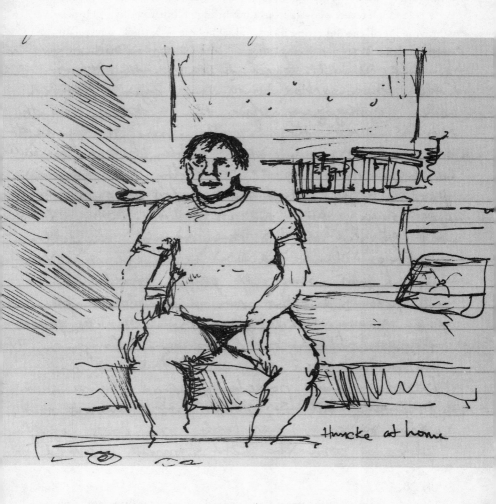

Huncke at home

as possible. We walked over the Brooklyn Bridge 'cause we were broke and Huncke borrowed five dollars from a neighbor in the building and slipped me one dollar saying, Here's a fin for ya.

At lunch recess we walked around through Chinatown with Huncke showing me all the old eating joints and telling me how the Chinese gamblers gamble all day and young whores'll come up and each gambler will take a break and fuck for a while—ten dollars a shot—and then return to the game. We shared a couple of oranges and a candy bar, and I bought him a Coca-Cola.

The sunlight was dazzling and beautiful, almost unreal against the shady streets of Brooklyn Heights—freedom in different measures after such a day. I was walking Huncke down State Street on the way home and I was slightly ripped from the smoke at Ondine's and Louis's, and that mixed with the weariness of the day brought the sunlight broken lenses and center crossroads traffic light sky into a swirl looking up. Feels real good, I said to him. Yeah man, it feels good, he answered.

Up at Ondine's Huncke asked me to come up 'cause he needed to hit on Louis for some of his piss. He had done two Valiums the night before court to get some sleep. He was real nervous and it didn't help. Wednesday he was going to have to give a urine sample at the methadone clinic and the only thing that should've shown was meth, not Valium. Louis was slightly ticked that Huncke had called me up to come down to the courthouse and didn't ask him to come. Huncke assured him that he did it only 'cause the wait would've driven him up the wall. I agreed knowing how it would've felt to Louis after the third hour. Louis could only piss a little into the bottle so I pissed the rest and a couple of drops of methadone was added to make it look cool.

July 28, 1977

Had a hopelessly beautiful dream—whole landscapes sliding by at rapid pace, retarded child imagery, lots of body movement, embracing. One old guy reappearing quite often in the frames, married and exuding all kinds of strange sexual energies. As soon as a guy appears in my dreams it seems I am faintly aware of the sexual currents inherent therein. Nothing terribly physical came of it all but the dream was one of the first I've had that when I woke up I recalled no violent fears or pressure of death and anxieties floating within it in the ropy passages of light and dark. It was like a night on the grand calliope of Breton's Amusement Park—something more soothing than the sexual Asbury Park of my seven-year-old mind.

July 30, 1977

What will I think of all this scribble ten years, thirty years from now in the change of history, where will Jim be or John or me in relation to all these activities? It's the starry mirror of the eyes' slow revolution to the impossible or fictional future then reeling back again to the past. FZZAMMM . . .

August 1, 1977

Met Huncke after work, dropped over to Arlene's house where he was staying. He was wrapped up in a bathrobe with white flesh coming out from the folds of cloth. He made us a vodka and grapefruit drink and we talked about Louis and the book. He said Burroughs and Ginsberg were to write notes for the back cover of the book and he would do the intro! I told him about Louis and Ondine trying to fix me up with the girl in Brooklyn. We were eating pitted black cherries and vanilla ice cream. I explained that I slept more with men than women at this point in my life. He said he understood and before I knew it he was calling it an evening. He repaid twelve dollars of the original twenty-two. I was under the impression that he owed me seventeen dollars, not twenty-two. Since he had no change of a twenty, he gave me twelve. Don't know if I'll see the rest and at this point don't care. I like Huncke both in an awestruck way: it's been great meeting him after reading stuff by and about him; and he is a kind of model in roles that I form my life after, things that directly influence me in directions. I also like him personally: his storytelling abilities are almost unmatched. But I'm not sure what he thinks of me. I'm sometimes like this naïve dude who's very easily taken, not by him necessarily but apt to be taken by anybody who has the desire to do that. I don't know if he looks at me that way, if I should assert myself at times and not do certain things. The things I see as going along to make a strong friendship, someone else could see as foolhardy or soft.

August 13, 1977

Jim McLaughlin, Louis Rivera, Dennis Deforge, and I went to a bar on Christopher Street. A miniature Ponderosa Ranch–style place with bleached cow skulls on the wall and a horse hitching post in the center of the room. Little lightbulbs flickering all over the place which was shadowy dark. One leather guy with muscle-bound chest and belly protruding from suit of leather with straps and white pants low sexy the belly kept moving through the crowd like one moves through a thick fog or water of a flood—looked like an SS agent with marble eyes and abandon wiped across his lips.

Met a guy there. Had noticed him looking in my direction but he didn't seem to want to approach with Jim, Louis, and Dennis around so when they split I stayed behind and talked with him.

We went for a walk around the Village near Soho—Houston Street—West 4th. His name was Ken Sterling. I liked him immediately, can't tell exactly what it was but a mixture of self-assureness. He was handsome in a way that people are handsome but not centered on it—one who doesn't spend time exercising good looks is extremely attractive in itself. We ended up at a café drinking cappuccino and a thunderstorm broke out. He finished college at nineteen. Just turned thirty years old. Was interested in linguistics, self-taught five languages, and currently studying Chinese. We went to his place in the West Village—a small two-room place with two small dogs, Electra and [?], a broken frame containing a print, an old washed color of North American Indian basket lid weaving of frog. Showed me a book on linguistics that had references to Aztec codices that had been banned by the Catholic Church. Burroughs had talked about such incidents in *The Job* and *Book of Breething,* I think. We lay down on a small mat/foam pad half under a desk and he read part of a poem by some guy twenty years old. It was quite good language smooth and rounded, rough in spots but not as hindrance. We turned out lights and made love without actually going the route for a fun time. The man is sensitive as hell. I can feel it through his touch and eyes and skin surfaces. Even without getting sexually involved to a high degree he was satisfying to be with. Someone I feel I could spend time with.

August 14, 1977

We woke up and walked the dogs and talked a bit then went to breakfast. We had omelets and coffee and I found a mosquito spread-eagled on the corner of my eggs and after hem and hawing we sent it back. The waitress came over and said, Oh I didn't realize they were even in season . . .

Ken would reach beneath the table and rub my leg or hand occasionally without much forethought—real natural and it was exciting. Never before have I been relaxed like that and able to accept the touch of a man who was also a lover in public—even beneath a table. I just didn't give a shit what anyone thought. It felt warm and nice. A friend of his came in who is into Gertrude Stein a great deal and was very gentle in voice and thought. Quoted lines from Stein that I could only paraphrase: A river in its rush and turn can become muddy but in its course of flowing the mud gradually settles and the water runs clear again.

This fella had recently broken up with a lover and said this sentence was like his life. He was all calm and had accepted the outcome of the relationship although the love pains were evident. Who can I read Gertrude Stein with now that we are no longer together? He had a marvelous voice for Stein's work.

Ken and I walked through the Village and Soho checking out bookstores. Ken bought a copy of Ezra Pound's *The Chinese Written Character as a Medium for Poetry* and another book on Chinese root segments of characters. He walked me to the subway and we kissed before parting. I literally moved home through fine gray filaments of sound and shapes, emotions running like flashes to past and projected future.

August 15, 1977

Ken called me at work. I had smoked a good deal with two other employees and was rather ripped. Felt tight in the head as I spoke to him because I had been thinking of him all day and really wanted to call but felt I should cool down and take it as it moves, like no frantic feelings, was excited hearing from him. Plans to get together Wednesday night. Will call him at eleven Tuesday night (tomorrow).

Stayed up last night until five A.M. rewriting "Cutting through the South," put in a quote from "Christ Is Alive in the Bum Sleeping in His Piss on a Sidewalk" by Plymell in the beginning under title of story. Made the story much more personal with prose—strange beautiful brain stuff—was half dead to finish it.

Got up at 8:30. Called work at 9:55. Was so tired and out of it that instead of squeezing my nose to pretend sickness I wrapt my hand around my throat, squawkin' . . .

Ken called. We talked for two hours on the phone. I was out of it having had no sleep at all. Hamburger was on the stove. We talked about hamburger burning up on a stove but I didn't get up to shut it off, kept talking about different stuff. I tried to explain the editorial qualities of REDM but fucked it up and blab-blabbed, felt terrible that I had come out sounding like personality judge. But it was really a fear that people would think that we have no notion of good writing 'cause some stuff was raw or rough, can't worry about it any longer really.

Met Ken in the evening, went to fantastic Animation Film Show. Ken touched me throughout the film putting hand over mine massaging it, his arm around my shoulders. The light on the screen alternately plunging the audience into discreet darkness and illuminating them/us. I felt a variety of changes in my head, at times extremely self-conscious of the moment other times feeling fine about it and glad of the changes I was working in.

We went to Sandalino's for salad and I talked a bit afterwards as we walked down Bleecker about what I felt as far as open affection in public places, that it was new to me, scared me a bit at times but that the embarrassment or fear was good for me to go through/handle/work with. Immersing oneself in one's fear produces opposite results—that area where it produces neither anxiety or ego-excitement. Don't know what the fuck to say about all this—

. . . While I searched continually to find the place and the formula.

September 10, 1977

Walked through Soho and over to Christopher Street, went to the big pier past the old truck lines and Silver Dollar Café/Restaurant where I spent many a night on the streets. Funny I see it all different—no longer a rush of (many) sad weird feelings hanging out in old areas. Feel real good today—kinda sad—good like a backwards glance over everything and seeing it all as okay and good vibes for the future it seems. Walked onto the pier and sat at the very end with my feet dangling like Huck Finn from his eternal raft with waves plash-plashing beneath every once in a while a great SWASH of water from a passing party boat or tug. Sunlight drift over New Jersey cliffs illuminates sparse architecture and great warehouses and piers and ships all shapeless from the blinding show of sun making it all look like India with orange postal card skies and you expect a huge herd of cows to be flat-walking over the river surface—where's the Taj Mahal!?

Came home and walked the Promenade a couple of times, the night sky clouds still slightly illuminated. Ghost whites beyond the night (sunset long gone) and met some fella named Bob walking through the streets a commercial artist and also artist/artist in the personal sense. He was out for a break in work—working in his own apartment/studio on some whiskey ads for Monday morning. We yakked awhile before retiring. He was wonderfully honest about his head and feelings—nice nice evenings of which I hope there will be more. I'm gonna get into weight lifting with him on Tuesdays and Thursdays 8–10 o'clock. He's got a healthy build and was

33

HUMAN HEAD II

What Will The Boy Become?

AT 15
STUDY & CLEANLINESS

AT 15
CIGARETTES & SELF-ABUSE

AT 25
PURITY & ECONOMY

AT 25
IMPURITY & DISSIPATION

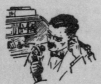

AT 36
HONORABLE SUCCESS

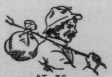

AT 36
VICE & DEGENERACY

AT 60
VENERABLE OLD AGE

AT 48
MORAL-PHYSICAL WRECK

JOURNAL © NEW YORK

previously like me in terms of skinniness so finally I'll have a chance to work out without hitting some gym.

Coming home on Montague Street. I stopped by the homemade ice cream parlor and ordered a vanilla-banana scoop with whip cream—sugar addict's delight. Real sweet girl behind the counter now recognizes me in fact two of them do. Said hi and all that and gave me a huge sundae for 85¢. NICE DAY—

September 19, 1977

SEEING MYSELF SEEING MYSELF SITTING BY AN OPEN WINDOW

When dawn comes on after a night that has spent itself by the window, dark ships ease into the frame of sky taking the place of clouds. Upside down they are sailing on and on toward an imagined horizon where the seekers of love stand to the side of the curtains peering out. There is great mystery, one of foreign soils and oceanic breath disappearing beyond the fine line of water and sky. We are growing steadfastly, fingernails and hair and subtle gray curves in the head. Lessons come in all forms from every direction, out on the bench by the river an old man sits swayed by neither water nor air, yet from this porthole several stories up I am seized by a continent of my own making.

Death and birth are just so much seawater floating around the curl of rocks and sand, there are pyramids and cliff dwellings that open their doors like great yawns to the upcoming sun.

How slowly we enter age and sleep, were it all a matter of putting one's head down and thought escaping like air from the insides of punctured tubes, movement would be a thin rose in the beaks of winged animals and today: a day of work and weariness would no longer be a necessity.

Food enters the mouth on the sharp edge of steel; it is not everything that we have bellies full or that our hair is shiny and combed. There are those of us that sleep well in doorways and on benches, not for reason or choice but because of the hard edge of vision in these times.

If I turned from twenty-three to eighty in the simple sway from window to bed what lives would remain in my heart, what answers to the questions of solitude and movement?

September 25, 1977

Gonna put together a collection of voices—overheard monologues or char-acter monologues that'll consist of junkies in a Chinese/American restau-rant in Frisco, junkie on 8th Avenue and 43rd, Arthur Treacher's Fish & Chips, Mike the bookstore guard, and the kid in Reno pickup truck, Huncke and others.* Illustrations will be photos of odd moments/people retreating into darkness/around corners/sliding off tables in old restaurants/back views/ views from the shoulders down.

[No date] 9:30 P.M.

Phone woke me at ten with Dennis on the other end. I was foggy and rub-bery I couldn't get my brains unscrambled. He was in Rahway, New Jer-sey, and was ill—possibly a flu—needed someone with a car to come and pick him up. I got the number of the pay phone he was nearby and prom-ised to call him back. Then sat with my phone/address book and called everybody to get a car. Most were not home and those who were didn't have a car at their disposal. Talked with Mom and she sounded slightly out of it—like pressure everywhere. She told me a story on young New York poets—with me, Dennis, and John in it, was going into Fordham Paper over the weekend. I called Syd in New Jersey; first time we talked in two years. I was afraid to call at first as I didn't know what was going on in his life, like maybe everything had changed and he was no longer interested in going out anymore. He was real happy to hear from me and we made plans to get together this coming Thursday. I realized how much I missed and love him. I would spend the rest of my life easy with that man if he weren't married and was open to a relationship—seriously. I grew through more heavy areas in my life with his aid than with anyone I know, and to renew contact with him was good.

*A chapbook of these monologues, *Sounds in the Distance,* was published in 1982 by Aloes Books, London, with a foreword by William S. Burroughs. In 1996, a more comprehensive volume of the monologues, *The Waterfront Journals,* was pub-lished posthumously by Grove Press.

I finally tried Laura and she agreed to come out with me to Dennis's spot and pick him up. I met her after a quick shower at Penn Central and we caught a bus out to her parents' house in Long Island. After arriving we discovered the keys were with her father at his job and we had to take a taxi over to pick them up. After that I called and said I wasn't coming to work till late and then we split. Made it out to Rahway hours later over the Verrazano Bridge through Staten Island and over the Goethals Bridge. Poor Dennis looked like Papa Grump with his thermal pants and undershirt. He looked healthy but moved around like he was tired and sick. We drove him home after loading the bike into the car and he gave yells of New York! God! I don't believe I'm home! etc. Laura let me drive for a period. Over the Verrazano I took the wheel and drove the rest of the way. Did okay although a slight mistake once. Sure I could pass the exam if I took it, ya know?

After Dennis went to sleep Laura and I stayed in the room adjacent to the kitchen and talked and listened to Handel, Wagner, and the Stones for a while. She reached towards me several times, wrapped her arms around me and I responded but held back as I felt it would be a bad thing for both of us if it went further. I don't want to start getting into a heavy relationship with her as there are too many complications in both our lives and though I do love her things won't be ironed out or balanced by that love. I called Jim and Louie and they told me to come right over so I walked Laura to the car and kissed her good-bye. She split to her parents' house on Long Island and I bought a bottle of wine and headed down to the party. The party was pretty nice. Jim and Louie had invited a lot of men all involved in the arts to a certain extent some maybe not but a diverse set of characters. I drank a couple of beers and didn't talk most of the evening as I felt removed from everybody. Don't know why, just felt slightly inhibited as I knew no one well enough and tire easily of bull-shitting conversations. I don't like to talk unless I mean what I'm saying, can't make small talk too well when I'm feeling down or inhibited so said little. Met this fella named John—the one person I did talk to for any period of time. He's an artist/painter, studies at the Art Students League, and works there making sandwiches once a week on Saturdays. We talked about hitchhiking and gradually I started feeling warm in my belly over him, wanted to tell him or say something to indicate what I was feeling but was unable to. Hope to see him again sometime.

October 6, 1977

Met Syd down near Port Authority on 9th Avenue in the rush of squallin' buses and fruit market pedestrian ballet. We headed for New Jersey and went to a motel/hotel across from the railroad tracks and across the street from mobile homes and trucks in the parking lot, etc. We talked about our past two years and I was glad we finally made it back together. It's amazing how he has grown in two years. I guess he's in his late forties or fifties and he made me kinda sad at times as I miss him and to hear some of the changes he and his family have gone through is amazing, all of them—the son shooting dope in the army, getting discharged, and eating himself into blimp size; wife getting operations on her ovaries, I think a hysterectomy; other children doing well. It was raining and we sat afterwards in a diner and ate lunch and talked about the city and its homosexual scenes, bars, etc. He drove me back later and I got out on the familiar spot on 40th and 9th to the side of the fruit stand, waved good-bye, and split across the honk snarlin' streets flap into the Port Authority building.

October 8, 1977

Went out to New Jersey and did the suburban trip for the day. It was pretty nice. First time I mowed the lawn in thirteen years or more I guess. Then we toppled the big weed tree in the front yard as it was dwarfing the huge red oak tree Dad had planted. I shaped the hedges square 'cause every other neighbor on the block had square hedges and I figured the house shouldn't look so conspicuous. Ha ha. So then me and Peter [David's younger half brother] got ripped on our asses. I toked some gold smoke in a homemade apple pipe Peter fashioned—real good idea. We got together with Billy Wayne and about six other kids and played nighttime basketball on an illuminated court in the woods with no lights around other than those of oc-

TIMES SQUARE PHOTO BOOTH

9/7 drifting viels & the sleeping mans desert
the earth suddenly stretched before the
sleeping eye — the vast curve line of vision
the earth curve; sleep of the traveler
easing into a sun filled crevice in the
clouds & those huge rolling sheep folds
of cloud-matter and a rose slash
spreading from the tip of some unseen
fire spreading over white lava — the
icey snow over drifting lakes — sunrise
over the seas brilliant whipped
formations that jut and curl and
form sheepskin textures — some vast
sleep world that jung would awake
in with harry crosby words of flying
the plane right into the sun echoing
in the memory and here it is foul
weather as the stewardess calls it and
the plane shakes til yr ears hum //
— Theres this baked look to the earth — the
shield curve is hard, cookin' — like asphalt
gleaming under sun — a few drifts of
clouds but the water takes on a
steely gray dead stone look — it stretches
behind the portals and the sun is too
intense to look at beyond that. Suddenly
its like seeing a strange series of
shapes in the distance — its areas
darker than the slant of ocean I've
been seeing for miles and miles
— they appear in the surface of
the ocean as if the surface of
the ocean were ice and these

casional car goin' on or off or by. Fuckin' stoned and played our asses off with great fun and glee. My perceptions were so strange—I'd be dribbling like a madman with quasi-fancy steps and think I see the basket a couple of feet behind me over my left shoulder so I'd spin around to shoot and blam! The basket would be twelve yards or more away. Then I'd go in for a layup shot and ZIP ZIP ZIP run like a drunken arrow towards the basket and do a layup and jump and sail and look up and there's the basket sailing by thirty-five miles an hour past and twist through (wangle) I'd pump a greasy shot in crazy and usually miss. Once in a while plip! It'd go in.

Before goin' to sleep Marion [David's stepmother] was complainin' about the work she's gotta do and how the kids don't seem to understand it all and she rambled on and on for about an hour and it was like she was realizin' how much she really loves the kids and how they try in certain ways and she ended with, They're pretty good kids, ya know? And I said, Well you're a pretty good mother, and she brightened up. It was a good moment for the two of us.

Before I went to sleep, I used the upstairs bathroom and in the floor were three bullet holes from where Dad shot a gun one night drunk. Made me feel strange and cold seein' it.

April 22, 1978

Dirk has a photograph that I wanna use for the cover of my monologues if they're accepted by any publishing group. He wants to do the layout for it (cover). The photo is a black–and–white of me with glasses off and hair slicked back. Linda and [Jan?] are in background fading away. It's a sharp high-contrast photo where I look (if nothing else) real striking slightly bizarre— not enough to distort what I feel about myself, and there's enough space for the title.

Harold is gonna lend me this typewriter next week to use for a week or two. I'm gonna type out all the monologues and send them off to Ferlinghetti at City Lights. Am thinking that that collection plus a couple of stories would be good as a book. Maybe photos by Dirk and Arthur Tress. Maybe no photos at all. Anyway it's all a major step as far as suddenly seeing enough good work by myself to send out to publishers—ain't worried about it being rejected as I'll put it out myself under the Redd Herring Press if no response from elsewhere. "Nevada Green," my story on the shotgun-wielding kids who picked me up outside of Reno for the twenty-seven-hour ride through cold mountains and dazzling heat, is shaping up slow but sure. Got lots of work in store for me there. Maybe send it to *Playboy* if I finish it and think there's a chance. Could use the money badly as Dennis says I'm all caught up in bills except the month's rent. And Red M/Zone party is coming up in two weeks. I need new fuckin' glasses, clothes, etc. Louis Cartwright's book needs $$ to be printed. It all brings a vast headache up to the shoulders. Phenas[?] wrote me from Crete and also Oxford, England. Things are going fine with him. I have to sit down and write him soon.

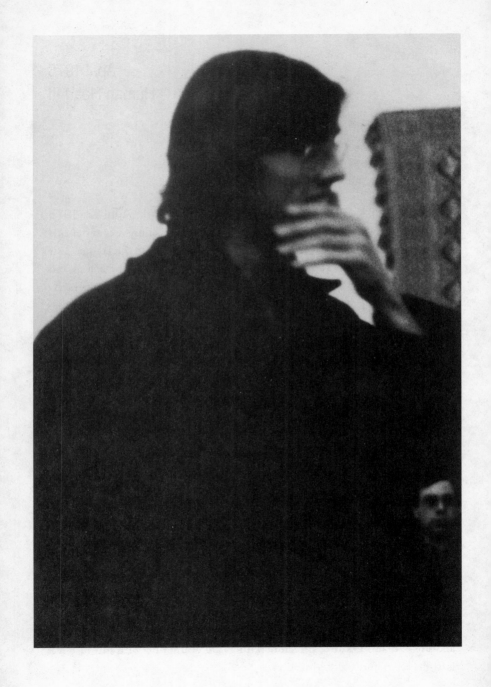

April 25, 1978

Met Syd tonight after work. We sat in a burger house and talked for an hour. I feel stilted in seeing him—seeing him means money for sex. I realize that when I met him one summer afternoon, I was fourteen and it was a sultry day—very little luck in hustling—the deaf-mute wasn't into going through fuck-fuck motions with his limp cock, and all the other people that had approached me wanted either film shots for ridiculous fees or heavy out-of-the-way (Far Rockaway or New Jersey) sex for five dollars. I was getting depressed not being in the money—John was with me and he had one fling which netted ten dollars and we both saw this guy checking us out and smiling from behind a newsstand, but the guy said he was interested in me. That was a bit of a rush. I was so used to men wanting John over me. We went up to the hotel on 44th Street or 45th up the rank rickety swaying leaning staircase paid seven dollars for a room and opened the windows to let the musty smell out. He was about thirty-seven and had a hard swimmer's body—very handsome—and I slowly undressed conscious of my white body, slim and angular against the dark colored walls. Set my clothes on the peeling hanger and we climbed into the cool sheets, the 8th Avenue wind from the river blowing the dirty curtains out over the Avenue—street sounds and prostitute clatter of heels mixed with traffic flowing in—a smooth and slow sex—laying back afterwards with thumping chests and sweat lining my neck and body warm breeze drying it all off—sheets moist and we talked slowly I had no idea of what price it all cost and he gave me twenty dollars. He was really nice, considerate, witty, and laid a calm hand to my chest for a while as he talked of sections of his life. We parted and saw each other regularly. At times his family was away at the shore and we would go to his huge mansionlike house in some rich section of New Jersey and in the backyard under the trees and stars lay out a blanket and made a wild love with fucking mosquitoes sending huge welts up my legs and sides and neck.

Seeing him tonight—years after all this was over—he had grown so much older—tight lines around his forehead and eyes—body kinda shrunken and bony. He talked about how his life was going (one of the monologues is his). I tried to explain to him what I was doing with my writing and art but realized that what I wanted to tell him was that I was successful—being published by this company and that company. But it wasn't possible because my writing is still being formed and there is no demand for it. The reason I wanted to tell him I was successful was to ease the concern on his part—to ease some kind of parental fears that I picked up from him. I told him this is what I was feeling. I told him that I didn't know what I wanted to do in my life other than paint and write. He suggested getting involved in some kind of company to pursue an interest and climb the ladder. I found it difficult to explain that I wasn't really at all concerned with notions of success in that sense—sure, I want to be recognized for what I do, but I couldn't get into the whole notion of competition, that if the by-product of my art acted as its own competition on the outside—on the street or wherever—fine, I have nothing to do with that. I could not, would not enter into the pushing of my work for competition's sake. I could not willingly get behind something I did and get into the dogfight of it all.

When we left the restaurant he stopped on the street and asked me how I was doing for money. I said I was desperate. He said How much do you need? and I couldn't say. Money from him, I haven't wanted money from him since I was eighteen. Never wanted to get paid for sex ever and yet I was broke, in debt for forty or fifty dollars plus rent and so he said how much? twenty dollars? forty dollars? I still shook my head, caught in the fucking nerve wires of resistance and need—opposites of the whole mess of what my life pointed to at that second. He said, One hundred dollars? Look, ya gotta give me some idea. Ya need rent money? What do you need? Tell me. I shook my head, I was stunned. He shoved one hundred dollars into my hand and I started trembling, crying, and shaking, the release of everything, relief of money needs, I stammered, said, Man . . . I don't know what to say, all these years I've wanted to tell you things but didn't know how. I mean, at this point I'm happy with what I'm doing in my life but when I was hustling, when I was in the Square at a certain point in my life, I really needed to connect with someone and you were really important then. You helped me through so many things, in ways you might not even be aware of.

He said, Well, that makes me feel really happy. And I shook his hand
and we said good night simultaneously and he turned and split and I turned
before he turned and I stood at the corner waiting for the light to change to
get across to the subway and was overtaken again and started crying.

May 2, 1978

Been working regularly on my monologues, still thinking out ideas for Artists Postcards series. The monologues are coming along fine—there's some
beautiful movement in them, genuine revelatory progression where character is revealing through conversation in an unusual way, where the thought
starts out in coffee shop banter and in progression parts the gray range letting
slip out some bleak or warm wing of the heart, the mirror behind the eye
slowly revolving. What excites me most is the potential of friends' stories for
monologues, got a beautiful one from Syd that came from my meeting with
him recently. It shows a tenderness mixed with ambiguity that is revealed
within the words—a sad sort of ambiguity/struggle with the spirit in between
social demands and physical/mental demands. Most of the monologues are
people once met and then left suddenly such as in car rides cross-country,
early-morning rail encounters, overheard coffee shop conversations, etc. They
are diverse enough to allow a continual transformation in the mind/eye. The
experience of them gradually broadens and hopefully in the end one will be
transformed in consciousness and in experience. Private personal glimpses into
the makeup of character, of America symbolized/represented by a handful of
characters. There's still an enormous amount of typing/editing in store for
monologues that were written down in loose form, editing of the sections
that slow down the emitting heart, the unnecessary sections of speech that
hinder the sections that contain the *glimpse*—the aperture of the dream.

May 25, 1978

Arthur called me this morning to say good-bye. He will be splitting soon to
go to California. He said Artists Postcards will contact me personally in a
month with the answer in regards to my postcard—the possible acceptance

of it for the show. He said he wrote me a letter and is mailing it today to me. I can't think of what it will contain—faint ideas that it may be in regards to our relationship. If I go to Europe in three months I won't see him and I don't know how I feel about that. I mean that I will miss him greatly, but I don't know if living in Europe will be difficult because of my loss of contact with him and all my friends. I'll be leaving so many people—my whole life behind me at that point as Europe represents total and uncommitted freedom—a drastic change in lifestyle and surroundings. I'll have no choice but to go ahead further into my life and explore possibilities as there will be no retreat into comfort of friends and lovers. I wonder if sex is possible with language barriers and secludedness of Normandy or offensive Parisians who won't speak to Americans, etc. It will be a confrontation of the senses.

August 27, 1978

Met a fella Friday night. Went into the Village after work and there was this character standing in front of B&S (Boots & Saddles) Bar and as I passed by him I realized that it was someone I had seen a number of times in Julius's but never spoke to—a fella who struck me as familiar in some nonspoken sense—like I knew him from somewhere but wasn't sure if he was just familiar from passing a number of times on the street or if he was from some place or gathering in the past. As I passed him it suddenly struck me that he was a man I went home with at age thirteen or fourteen and that was up on 58th Street near the park. The fella back then had had a swimmer's body— the first very handsome guy I'd ever gone to bed with. That time I was into going downtown to Times Square a lot. We had met in front of the theaters on 42nd. He took me for a soda in the seafood place on 43rd Street, and we ended up going to a friend of his house and makin' it. I didn't ask for money at that time—the second time I ran into him I went with him and he and I made it again in the same apartment and then as I was getting dressed I mentioned to him that I usually asked for money and that I didn't want to in his case but did he think it was possible to give me a few bucks because I was hungry. He said he never picked up hustling kids but sure and threw me a couple of bucks—never saw him again but thought about him as I was growing up—those savage déjà-vu strikes in the center of the heart when there's that odd recall of a man you have lain down with—where has he gone to?—what changes in the visual sense. Here I am ten years later completely away from that whole intense neon scene of the square—

He turned his head as I passed. I turned and looked at him for a moment trying to remember and place him ten years later, aging and all. I

47

walked on to the corner and hung out there for a while and soon he came up. I explained to him where I felt I knew him. He had indeed lived on 58th Street ten years ago, had friends who had apartments on 58th Street, but he didn't remember me. We exchanged phone numbers and I split, planning to get photos from Dirk and see Brian. As I left and headed toward Dirk's house I realized how much I must have changed visually for this guy not to remember me. When I met him his features were of a thirty-year-old, I guess, and pretty much formed (so I could recognize him years later). Yet I had changed considerably. In my wallet I had a photo from a Times Square photo machine and had I pulled that one out he probably would have had a start.

Later on Friday night I met a fella in Julius's bar. I saw him immediately after getting a coffee and walking near the front door of the place. His name was Phillip and he'd just returned from a trip out to Montana where he'd camped out and hiked through national parks of the nearby states. I liked him at once real friendly fella, smiling a lot, and I got an incredibly positive sense from him. He told me how he had broken up with a lover he had for eight years and took that Montana, etc. trip to get some deep thinking done, to get further in touch with himself. I thought about it and was touched and amazed at the thought of eight years with a fella. He seemed like someone one would want to spend one's life with on first meeting—I get carried away, huge tumble rush of glad-in-the-boots-up-to-the-eyes feeling, like meeting him was this big relief that came winging over my shoulders into my chest removing all the hectic thinking and musing and pondering of the last month. I told him a bit of my travels out in Montana, descriptions we offered to each other were immediately recognized and there was this toss-of-the-head mobile-shoulder-yah-yah of agreement about the whole sense of western country space beauty stillness and the giant image of rolling earth before one's eyes. He asked me if I cared to go back to his place and smoke—Oh man did I! He explained to me his work, how he never had been inclined toward working in the arts, trying expressions through a great deal of school and then he got into contact with clay and that's where it started—

he's been successful in his growth in the medium—getting accepted in some ceramics organizations or groups that were difficult to get into. I felt glad for him 'cause, as he explained, getting accepted validated the works that he had done. I understand what that is, it's like my manuscript being held at City Lights—if they or someone else publishes it it'll be like a big push in the direction of my work, support from those you respect.

He showed me these beautiful pieces, like a show-and-tell, he said, the progression of his work over the last four or eight years. All throughout his house he had beautiful objects: tree growths/limbs/rocks/a huge wasp nest—his lover had gotten it for him. He became animated and excited over showing me the stuff and I was swept back, taken full force by his excitement, his great eyes so full of energy from form and design and the sense of touch. His ceramics were beautiful, a great deal of sensitivity in them. The thing that really hit me was his interest in nature—it brought me back fully into a huge cargo of senses and memory, the whole denial of the love for nature that had taken place from so much city living, that whole period where I ceased drawing and my desire for writing precluded just about every other sense, my many animal books down in some faraway basement uptown.

We made love and it was exhilarating, the passion something I had not felt to that degree in some time, mostly because of the concern over all events transpiring in last two or three months. He talked about *Findhorn Gardening*—have to read the book—it made him aware of the presence within a forest of all these living things. Sort of like an entity of its own. I didn't want to leave but had told Brian I would see him later. I left around 2 A.M. and went home. I've been kind of in a dreaming daze from all the thoughts produced in that meeting with him and have not stopped thinking about him since Friday night. We might get together Monday night. I hope so as I'd like to see him again before I go. We made plans to correspond with each other while I'm in Paris and Normandy. I feel kinda confused 'cause my emotions have run away into an area of little control where I hardly know the fella but feel such a great deal for him. He's a teacher in a school that has a semiexperimental setup, a setup that every school should have. His contact with the kids is on the same level both ways: he's in touch with a great deal of their ideas and needs and desires, and he teaches arts and

sciences, tries to merge the two, which by the looks of his work he suc-
ceeds greatly, by furthering the textures of nature in the surface of clay, always striving to bring it further along.

August 29, 1978

We drove onto the upward ramp and into the second-story platform of the
garage, hunted awhile for a space, found it and parked. We walked down
the ramp, he with his hat on, the fine drizzle sparking the night, and my
feet were fluid. I could walk for years just thinking about possibilities and
the endless listening which somehow became so important to me, like I
wished I knew him for all of his thirty years just so that I could say or respond to what he was talking about in the way that would most put his
mind/heart at ease. I could see how much he was troubled by it all, the
story of homosexual lifestyles and drawbacks that could very well be spoken similarly by Dennis, Harold, myself, and Brian, and so many other people
I have known. What knocks me away is that there are all these men who
feel similarly but they never find each other or partners in each other. Here
I feel like I could spend a great deal of the time with Phillip but am struck
by the seeming senselessness of this thought because I met him now for the
second time and I'm channeling all this emotion and thought to him—how
right is all this? how possible for it all to work out someday in this lifetime
for all of us? But it isn't senseless in that I do see the heart of men by and
through their eyes, that space of liquid in the aperture of the head that re-
veals energy and life and sensitivity, all the positive energy rushing from
him in the things he desires for his own mind (the fool who left him after
eight years).

I gave him a long massage and from his head to his toes, kneaded and
rubbed to work the tension out—what feelings I try to move through the
tips of my fingers. We went to bed without having sex and I really didn't
care, sleeping next to his warm body was enough and when I woke the
seven times during the night startled awake from high-strung senses from
realizing I would not see him again after tonight I wanted the night to move
so much slower wanted the breath to leave me drifting when dawn finally
came through the windows drifting in some nameless sleep that none of us

know until that point where we become speechless and unconcerned with the journey of our bodies and environments. A separation from the senses so as not to feel the loss. When I woke in the morning the sun was filling the courtyard and windows painting a fine white line across the sills, and I had a great need for a cigarette, went into the kitchen and leaned against one of the counters among the various smooth/rough instruments, bowls, seated objects fashioned from clay, and there were rusks of binded husks from wheat and big seedy bulbs of dead sunflowers and a cuckoo clock and a pastel of a forest and in among all that I recalled with a slow drawing on the cigarette the night before and the emotions of the two of us towards sleep the continual brush of lips and hands and the warmth of skin, the surfaces of our two bodies instilling so much love and confusion in this weary and runaround heart of mine, and then I went back to bed and climbed in under the covers and put my arm across his smooth chest and slowly drew it back and forth and slowly he responded and I slipped further beneath the covers touching his chest with the tip of my tongue and running it around his breasts and down his smooth sides and across his belly into his legs and took him into my mouth and he reached down taking hold of me and there followed a slow sex that turned frantic as he crossed the threshold of sleep and we both came simultaneously and I wearily dropped down into the blankets my heart like some red horse galloping in the nervous arena of my chest and lay there looking around the room—on one wall the tied stalks of Montana wheat from where he drove and drove and drove through endless roads past endless fields of rich green wheat in the summer heat and down there somewhere in that western country he stopped his Volkswagen and grabbed a handful because it startled and amazed him into some kind of dream state.

After a while he got up and made coffee and toast with some Norwegian goat cheese and let Willow his pet rabbit out for a walk and I remembered how he named his Volkswagen Huck and how with the letter to him explaining as much of my senses from our contact and the piece of driftwood in a box waiting to be brought to his doorstep tomorrow morning I have this sad heart because of what might well have been, no longer possible, and now what might possibly be affected by this letter, this gift but regardless, I give it up to him with a true feeling in my heart, a real sense expressed and I don't think negativity could possibly come from up-front emotions regardless of the range and the disquieting fact that we hardly know one another at all.

September 1, 1978
Harriet Tubman Park

Okay, so I'm in front of the Chinese Laundromat where my clothes are undergoing tumble, morning with clear light, sifting through last night's dead mysteries, a coolness to the hot breeze within my cheeks and arms. Chance has taken another turn making me undecided about whether I subscribe to chance. Ha, don't have a choice it seems but were it to turn in the directions it does at these times I may well get over all formal mental expectations for the cranking whirl of this great planet and throw myself back into the heaping whirlwind of mobile shift philosophies—no denigrating stud-shoe dance in particular, but let it be as it be—don't struggle.

Phillip called the store yesterday around one o'clock, my stomach was like a clutch stuck in shifts. We made plans to get together for lunch down in the West Village around Sheridan Square. I was down there around two, he showed up and we went over to Bleecker and West 4th bar-restaurant and sat outside in the cool wind—me with a mushy bowl of chili, just 'cause it's cheapest on the menu, and two coffees. He talked back and forth with me but I was in back of my mind waiting for a word about my letter and suddenly he leans forward and says the letter was beautiful—he'll be glad to be caretaker for shelf figure piece I gave him. I'm startled, all relief coming out the back of my head mixing with West 4th Street wind, so much relief, so worried was I that he'd be frightened by my letter. I couldn't even remember what exactly I'd written, I mean if tone was frantic-adolescent, but straight from the heart. I could hardly eat. He seemed slightly uncomfortable and we got into such heavy subjects—parents, alcoholism and parents, Al-Anon (its good points), therapy, etc. When we left we walked down to Houston Street and he outlined children's book he was writing and I asked if I might have a crack at illustrations. He said he'd send pages to Paris for me.

If anything is difficult to do it's writing about someone you care for a great deal while all emotions and projected dislikes, etc. take their places in the shifting balancing act for more clear perspective. I see that all I've written this morning awakens different strong senses in eye and heart and am not sure where my sense of self is drifting.

So we say good-bye and he tells me: I won't wish you a good trip yet 'cause I'll probably see you over the weekend, if not I will speak to you (he canceled his trip to Montauk). So I return to work, arms and legs tense, feeling relieved but unhappy that I was in such a state of mind as to not be able to relax and enjoy fully the get-together. The call was so sudden and the anxieties of whether I'd done silliness again in my life—big risk of the heart. Jimmy and the people at the store bought five bottles of champagne and a big cake and six joints and everybody got blasted and started running around and cracking jokes and monologue routines. Jimmy said, Nobody wants any more cake? and slammed his face into the cake and walked around the store all globby, cake cream filled in the pockets of his eyes, and then Ricky pummeled his own face into the cake and there were a lot of hoots and hollers and racing around transfixed customers and the air drifting down from the office onto the floor reeked of champagne that foamed all over the tables and cake smeared on the floors and smoke of grass wafting in and out making it all smell like weird vinegar fifty years old open on shelf in some hot kitchen. I got real weary and talked with everyone in good-bye tones and finally at 9:45 when store was closed down stood outside Madison Square Garden and the whole thing hit me hard—I was leaving. I felt uncertain about Phillip, how he felt, and so I went down to West Village and ate a sandwich at Sandolino's. The waitress there—the one who has a new wave sense and French accent whom I've gotten to like a lot for all her darned words and perceptions, like the time Brian and I walked in there buzzing from two massive peyote milk shakes and I went to use the bathroom and she went up to Brian and hit his shoulder with the back of her hand and said, Psst, whatcha guys on? She's real nice to me and I refrain from saying, Hey I'm leaving the country possibly for good and I'm gonna miss ya. After the sandwich I check paperback corner for Krishnamurti books, they're out of stock on 'em. As I'm leaving the store I think of how it is that in working on making contact with something I may run into them or someone like that, but in the lamplit street rush of outta-towners here for Labor Day weekend I don't see him, I rush past the darkness of Sheridan Square Park and down a couple of streets to Julius's for coffee, maybe for sexual contact. I'm feeling a lot of bumming in my head. I order coffee at the busy counter and looking over I see Phillip sitting there. I cover my face in mock embarrassment but he looks right past me three times. Finally he sees me and we get over to the bar and talk. He says he was gonna go either (1) to a movie, (2) to the Al-Anon meeting, (3) to the baths tonight. He chose the meeting and we talk for a while. I finally can't take it and tell him I was feeling funny about the letter, how it might've been taken. He says, Hey, look, I'm telling ya I thought the letter was beautiful. I'm gonna keep it 'cause of that. I understood what you were saying, how our meeting woke up all these things in you. Ya can't go back into the past and try to figure out my thoughts or anybody's thoughts, like did he take it this way or that way 'cause it doesn't matter, it doesn't make a difference how someone perceives something like that. You wrote it and said what ya had to say and what I take it as isn't your responsibility. If I take it wrong or other than you intended then that's my problem if it's a negative reaction that results. It's just something that you can't do anything about. That's the way it goes and you shouldn't worry about it. If it's disappointing then still you've done what you thought was right and that's all you can do. When I first read the letter I went, Uh oh . . . Oh no . . . and then I said, Lemme read this and take it just as it is and not add anything more, not read my own ideas into it. And I realized that it was beautiful—it came from this core within you, straight from the core, and that's really good—

September 4, 1978

Charlie Plymell called this morning. Somehow he had gotten my number. He said he received the manuscript, he thought it was great, that it had chances for international publication, over in Europe. He had no money, was trying to figure out how to get tomorrow's groceries, otherwise he would publish the book himself, he felt it was that good. He said that Ferlinghetti was sometimes "stupid on these things," talking about publishing my book and how his book *Last of the Mocassins* has sold out and something about getting 250 dollars for the run and how he could have gotten 2,000 dollars for 500 copies but he fucked it up. He said that he didn't know my chances for getting the book published, but that it was great. He recommended a book that I should read: *Waiting for Nothing,* by Kromer (Hill & Wang). He said Sylvia, a woman who owns a bookshop and helps edit *Gasolin,* would probably like some parts for *Gasolin*—check it out. Gotta write him from France.

I called Dolores [David's mother], and she said she had been to a medium and the medium got in contact with a British fella, a spirit, and that the fella, when asked about me said, Oh no oohhh . . . the stubborn one! He said that I had to realize, it is not a crime not to know everything. He said that I would be successful in my art and writing, that I would be healthy all my later life and I would get my hot temper under control after a while.

He also said that Dad realized what he had done and that he was sorry for it and that he was at peace.

●Auto Noir●
l'an de le cheval
[JOURNAL]

SEPT. 14. 78 PARIS ∾ NORMANDY OCT 18TH .78

°THIS JOURNAL IS DEDICATED TO BRIAN BUTTERICK AND
THE YOUNG TEXAN IN THE WEST COAST MIDNIGHT HOTEL°

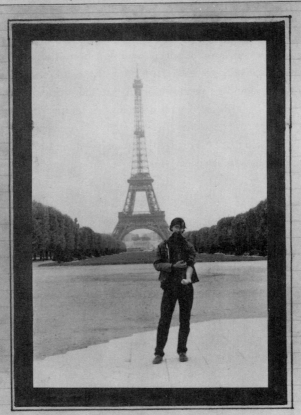

horse

September 16, 1978

J.P. [Jean Pillu, Pat's husband] drove Pat and I to the doctor's on the left bank of the Seine. J.P. waited across the street in a bistro while we went inside. Pat was gonna have an IUD inserted because she wants to get off the pill. I went into the outer doctor's office while she explained the problems I was having with a rash and prescription. The doctor took me inside and examined me and then took Pat inside for the insertion of the IUD. The door remained open and after a couple of minutes she started yelling in pain—it was terrible. I thought of how terrible it is that women undergo this sort of shit for men. It's something I would never say to her as I feel she might get upset. I might not have any business saying it anyhow. But I remembered when Jez and I were in our relationship, how she was gonna do the pill or some other method but I insisted she not, that I would do rubbers. What had upset me was that she immediately assumed the responsibility of taking precautions. I think it is the responsibility of the male since it comes down to the fact that all of the options available to women seem to endanger their own health. It's complex, it's just that when it comes to insertion of foreign objects or medicines I would rather undergo the slight decrease in sensitivity wearing a rubber than the woman do that to herself.

Pat screamed out a few times and started talking to the doctor about how she was going to faint, and how very much like her adolescent periods the pain was, how she would have cramps so severe when she was younger that she would faint or get extremely nauseous. She yelled some more and I found myself tying my fingers into knots feeling what she must have been going through. I wished J.P. was there to hear. Pat went home afterwards

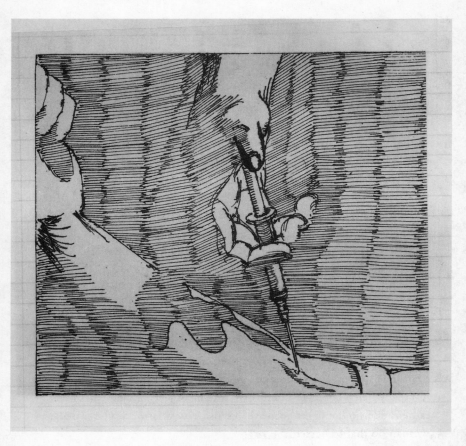

and took a painkiller and went to sleep. J.P. and I went to the Marcel Proust
Flea Market to check out clothes, etc. I found a couple of books that I've
either wanted to read or have never seen or heard of. One was called *Cut
Up or Shut Up,* a book by Carl Weissner and two other fellas with ticker
tape by W. S. Burroughs. The other book was John Rechy's *Numbers,* a
book Brian had recommended.

J.P. and Pat bought me a typewriter for my birthday! J.P. and I found
it in the Proust Flea Market. It is an Underwood machine in great condition—type lined perfectly, all letters clear as new, and a handsome fuckin'
machine. Now I can write poems and start on the novel and finally write
decent letters to friends. (Ah, but the fuckin' postage!)

So now I'm back in bourgeois St.-Germain, cruising grounds for
prowlers/pickpockets/homosexuals/fire-eaters/jugglers and the famous
Ratman who a year ago gave some woman a heart attack with his live rats
on strings—now he's been reduced to plastic rats by the police. Ate ravioli
in my Italian restaurant with the waiter who reminds me of Jerry Leo—
he looks like a French Bruce Springsteen. Real handsome in hustler tight
pants.

September 17, 1978

Had an incredible lunch with J.P.'s mother, sweet woman white/blond
haired, très French looking much like Giselle, Dolores's friend from Paris
who dug clams in the briny mint green surf of Atlantic City, New Jersey,
with us in swimsuits back sometime in '64–'65, a hot summer before I got
into the Times Square scene and all that hot sooty neon and hotels.

So she made potatoes and garlic, watercress salad, and veal and string
beans and afterwards we went out in the car. She was powdered up and
lipsticked and in a white suit we drove to le château du Versailles and strolled
to one of the entrances of the gardens.

We walked around the gardens and over to the fountains with les
poissons rouges! Les poissons rouges! Like a Ferlinghetti poem I read years
ago when in the silence of the November dusk when no one was watching
a shadow turned its head.

- I'm splashing water on it to see the band colours clearly

a snake trying to eat all the animals in a pet shop – it goes to eat some small birds that are loose – they can't get away – they go to fly but descend instead of ascend.

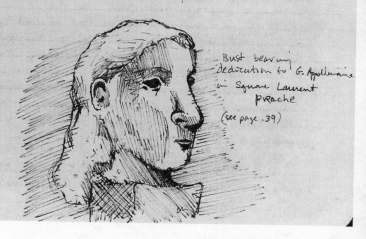

" THE ROLE OF THE ARTIST IS TO BECOME INHUMAN; HE MUST LOOK FOR WHAT IN ART HAS "MOST ENERGY;" SCORN FACILE CHARM, LEAP FORWARD AND ASSERT THE CLAIMS OF POETRY AND PAINTING TO EXPLORE THE WORLD OF THE FUTURE, CLAIMS WHICH ARE PRIOR TO THOSE OF PHILOSOPHY, PSYCHOLOGY, AND SCIENCE. "

– HENRY PEYRE / GUILLAUME APPOLLINAIRE

– Bust bearing
dedication to G. Appollinaire
in Square Laurent
Prache

(see page .39)

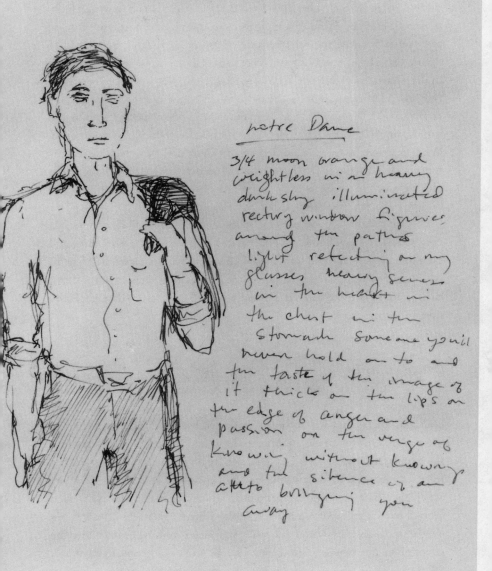

notre Dame

3/4 moon orange and
weightless in an heavy
dark sky illuminated
rectory window figures
among the paths
light reflecting on my
glasses heavy senses
in the heart in
the chest in the
stomach Someone you'll
never hold on to and
the taste of the image of
it thick on the lips on
the edge of anger and
passion on the verge of
knowing without knowing
and the silence of an
atteto bringing you
away

September 19, 1978

Got my haircut today. (Pat and I took the metro—easy-riding rubber-wheeled trains in huge tile stations with curved walls.) I had to wear a fluffy pink robe because mostly women went to the place. Funny, my intense reaction to wearing the robe because of its pinkness, don't know what I fear in that. The haircut was nice. Went to St.-Germain after lunch and wrote in my journal at a table at Café Flore, read sections of John Rechy's *Numbers,* a good book though I feel I write much better and that there's a lot I could do with the material had there never been books written by him, the stuff I come in contact with. He is good at times, very dry observatory eye. Wonder where he's at now, somewhere in his forties? Wonder if he'll commit suicide rather than face the decline of his body, that which he loved so fucking much in the pages of his novels, his obsession with the self, affirmation through others desiring him.

Noticed the businessman who speaks good English and French—looks very American. Saw him last night. He sat next to me at the Café Flore and I felt him cruising me and tonight saw him there with what seemed like his wife and kin. He looked up and regarded me with interest, with my hair cut I'm looking more intense especially when wearing my blue corduroy shirt almost black.

October 8, 1978

Stare up at the lonesome night with its irregular stars and mirror of vast calm over upturned eyes. A blond young man in a bright white shirt and fine body pushing against his clothes was pursued by most of the characters in the garden. He cruised me but I turned away and ignored him walking into the circular mound of earth and grass and lay on my back checking out the solar system 'cause I didn't wanna feed his ego as he was stunning—desperate characters crashed into trees and bushes pursuing him. Later as I walked around he was still cruising me and finally I made it with him. It was très gentle and at the same time frantically passionate and we did it under the cover of an area where there were no men—orgasm so explosive I almost fell to my knees. Before parting I traced an *X* over his heart in a kind of quiet gratitude for the fast sexual act and the intensity of his senses so apparent in the encounter and to take the place of my inability to communicate the desire for an encounter away from the park and in the warmth of a home and bed, the communication that isn't quite there in outlaw sexual encounters no matter how much sense is transferred. He smiled and grasped my waist and arm in a quick hug and I trailed off across the cobbles into the taxiing night looking for transport.

October 16, 1978
[Copy of letter sent to Christian Bourgois Editeur]

Dear Editor,

I am twenty-four years old and have lived on and off in New York City for twelve years. In the last four years I've spent a great deal of time hitchhiking and freight-hopping across the highways and folds of America, and have spent a good deal of that time living around the back streets of various cities. From this period I've collected a series of monologues—sections of conversations from junkies, prostitutes, male hustlers, truck drivers, hobos, young outlaws, runaway kids, criminal types, and perpetual drifters. These monologues were not written down with the aid of any tape-recording device but were the bare sections of one-way conversations that I retained in memory till minutes, days, or weeks later when I would write them down in journals and scraps of paper and in letters to friends around the U.S. They contain bits of road philosophies, accounts of street life & road life, anxieties of America's young who live outside of society, and sections of word-flights from the lips of characters who needed to articulate for themselves and me what their lives have been composed of. I merely served as a filter for all of this. This collection is called *Sounds in the Distance: Thirty-eight Monologues from the American Road*. I recently erased my own borders and have come to live and write in France. I stay on and off in Paris and Normandy with family. I have a copy of this manuscript with me and am interested in submitting it for your consideration. Charles Plymell (editor of Cherry Valley Editions) should be sending me the name or names of persons who might be interested in translating the book. In the meantime

I would like to know if you are interested in looking at the copy I have and if not would you have an idea of a publishing company I might send it to as an alternative?

Thank you—

David composed many letters to his mother, Dolores, with whom, by this time in his life, he had very little direct contact. For the most part it is presumed that these letters were not posted. In fact, by the time David was featured in a cover story for The Village Voice *in 1990 by C. Carr, his mother was completely out of touch with him, and from this article she learned for the first time that he had a successful career as an artist, and that in his work he revealed and explored the meanings of being HIV-positive in this culture.*

October 17, 1978
Sections of letter to Dolores
RE: JOURNAL WRITING

Keeping some form of journal is important for both the practice of writing and the slow articulation of thoughts. You grow so much over a period of time in writing things down, you don't have to necessarily keep a daily journal, it can be composed of ideas, plans, future projects, emotions, things on the mind, places to visit for the purpose of photography, what in certain photographs excites you (when you get into this it becomes very helpful for learning how to articulate your senses and also creates a definition of what you are trying to do or what inspires you and from there more ideas spring), what mannerisms or qualities people have that you respond to, why this kind of light as opposed to that kind of light is more appealing. Continually define for yourself what you sense. Most of us respond to or are struck by things first on an intense emotional level and though that is important still it is better if we try to define the senses, for then we learn what our critical outlook is composed of, why it responds to certain things rather than others. We in effect learn so much more about ourselves and also map our elusive selves . . . and a sense of groundlessness, of diverse chance. I try to accustom myself to this sense: trust it and accept it without resistance, as change keeps our senses alive, keeps us coasting and viable human beings . . .

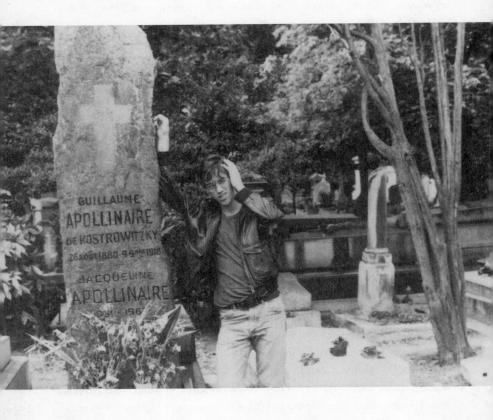

I may burn out before long but in the meantime I go on . . . like sometimes I'll be hit with a feeling, I stop everything I'm doing and with cigarette in hand I'll pause long enough to be overwhelmed at the enormity of what my life is or has been, all of it suddenly catching up like a huge line of shunted railroad cars to the main engine . . . the realization of it is not slow and does not give me a chance for adjustment but rather it comes rocketing out of the night with an earsplitting jar—crashing into my head and heart . . . and I'll have to shut my eyes and push the entire image away so that I can breathe again, because it overwhelms me so severely that all the sense that I've made of it, all the reasons for it being the way it is, suddenly become quite mean-ingless in the face of the knowledge that I'm just one of the millions or bil-lions of characters rushing, spilling, groping, pushing, shouting, laughing, crying, dying, heaving, tumbling, gesticulating, and clambering through the air and space of what we have come to call earth and body, the marketing rocketing meat-machine motion, each one of them similarly intent on finding purpose or creating change. I don't think I could ever come up with a word or phrase that could define the emotions that arise at that moment other than that it's utterly frightening and enigmatic . . .

RE: THE "VEIL" SHE SPOKE OF BETWEEN US IN OUR LIVES

I might as well go one step further. In your last letter you spoke of a veil having been between us for a long time. Aside from the things which I need to keep private, the aspects of my life which are intensely personal and which I share with few people, there are areas which I have felt unable to share with you because of the fact that you are my mother (I hope that doesn't sound like I'm saying it's a fault). I mean that I have in my head an idea of what it would be like to be a parent and to see your child grow up, to see him grow up outside of the personal hopes or expectations you might have formed for that child and I see the chances for both unexpected pleasure and equally unexpected pain within the eyes of the parent as he or she watches the child moving about (the child being four or twenty-four). So far my life has been filled with a variety of situations and circumstances where I have ended up roving through scenes that are very removed from scenes most people commonly go through and as a result of this I have developed a keen

THERE'S A VAGRANT ON THE TRACKS

VERSE 1   MAN TRANSMITS

figure to stone

~~line~~ line to paper

when he's all alone

its like a telescope eye

a fragment of the sky

a slice of the moon

like a heart in ruin

VERSE 2   its a seacoast secret

a mirror in the sand

its a lifeline of a stranger

in a polished hand

thats lookin for controls

to a heart fulla holes

thats the mammal crime

in the silent skyline

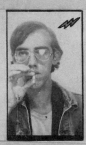

– a pale whisper; a sound of homelessness in the throat.

(from airmail envelope writ in gloom punk darkness by the spittin fountain after the encounter) Jardin des tuileries

we cansee a dead man die oblivion comes only once in a lifetime: photo of man falling on tracks
but

TALENT IS COURTESY WITH RESPECT TO MATTER; IT CONSISTS OF GIVING SONG TO WHAT WAS DUMB.

             – JEAN GENET
             (THIEFS JOURNAL)

sense of awareness of the darker areas of society and its characters. I have
also developed my own sense of moral outlook that has been fused with the
outlook I have learned from social institutions like school, etc. I end up
having more of an acceptance of characters and styles of living that seem to
go against the established order of the church and society—these people and
the ways in which they live do not frighten or disturb me. At times I find
myself picking up some of the things I see and trying them. It is in the very
midst of this that I see chance for pain in you if you were to see this happening or if I were to tell you. Not only that, but there is a tremendous
amount of confusion in these times when all that I have been taught col-
lides with what I am experiencing . . . sometimes things are very exciting
or pleasurable and all my past teaching from school, etc., tells me that it is
neurotic to experience or even enjoy such a thing, thus a confusion comes
about as I rapidly try to assimilate the experience and decide for myself (regardless of what I've been taught) what it is I feel in regards to that experience. Now to place that confusion in your hands or heart could very easily
create a concern or pain when connected to your possible hopes for me. I
couldn't chance that or I should say, I wouldn't. I think every person has
this vacant space with his or her parents and it is not meant to exclude because of lack of feeling but on the contrary because of love for the parent.
So when you experience this veil it is not because I am intentionally ex-
cluding you; it is because I must, it is because I, as the person moving through
the experience, will almost certainly see it differently from you, as you are
unable to see it below its face value (I am not casting doubts here as to the
quality or openness of your perceptions, just that in certain areas that I move
there are great amounts of socially produced misconceptions and you cannot help but pick up those misconceptions in order to try to understand the
action, we all do this to a degree). I don't think anybody is able to see more
deeply below the surface of the experience than the person going through
it, so therefore I might be past the experience and moving through the stages
where I decide if it's valid for myself and worth going on with while you
are still seeing the visible aspects of the thing and quite possibly being upset
by it. It's funny because my writings reflect a great deal of these experiences

and awarenesses and you can't help but at one time or another see and read those writings . . . so I am always aware of the eventual possibility of your reading about my life or senses of it upon publication and it's strange to wonder what your feelings or reactions will be. Though I am concerned about them still I must continue to write what I feel is important or necessary. So as usual I must just grin and bear it and hope for the best . . .

This journal is dedicated to Jean-Pierre Delage

[No date]

Met with Jean-Pierre sometime in the evening around eight o'clock at the St. George metro station. Me, standing around with fists in lonely pockets, wondering if I got times screwed up maybe I was supposed to meet him around six or seven instead and all other sorts of last-minute nervousness one has when meeting with a new lover: all notions of love and romance for the future perfecto are thrust and projected and yet there's that minute fragment of fear that it will all be swept away in a strong wind my real sense of the lover waiting is the Sisyphus stone poised for an interminable moment caught between the push upwards, the elevation, and the gravity pull downwards as in unending search, that flight of hands beneath the cloth of the trousers in the hidden pockets wondering if that rush of heart-speed will once again face an empty bed of noncommunication . . . more days of sub-vocal speech to whirl and drift 'cause there's no one there to talk with . . . He shows up and says, Ah ah I'm sorry I'm late and with all the cool of Marlowe I shove my sleeve up to reveal my bare wrist and take note of the time on my imaginary watch and say, Aw no you're not at least not by my watch, and he laughs and with a slim hand propels me along with him in his chugging vehicle and we're off into the Parisian night talking madly in half English half French between gesticulations and sign languages composed on the spot. I'm learning the famous French sign language originated not by the French but by lonesome men and women of foreign countries meeting in the night and trying to erase the silence. We head over to St.-Germain

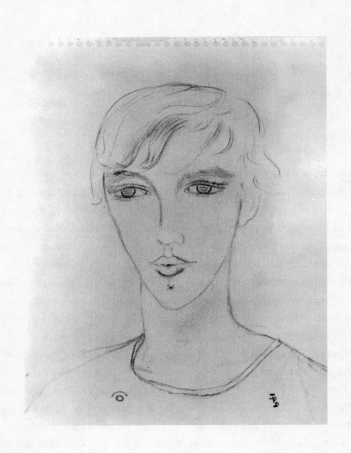

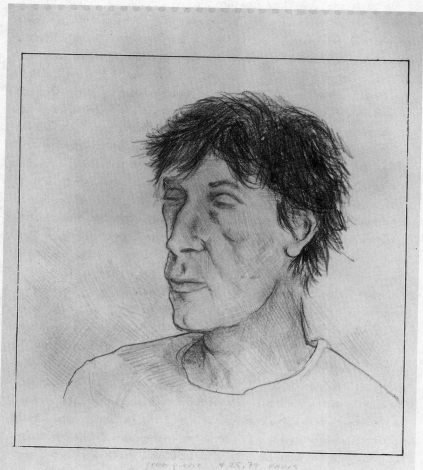

jean-pierre 4.25.79 PARIS

to a tiny restaurant where just an evening before some ratty dog jumped out from the door as I passed and yap-yapped at my retreating mysterious figure in the night causing me to turn and fake a Frankenstein movement at it just to send it into a nervous tither: giving it a chance to work out a year's supply of anxious vocals . . . But tonight the dog was gone and the place was a huge rosy kitchen of French characters like Mom's dining room and all these lovely people all chewing away at various foods and yak-yakking and looking up as we walk in and some young woman in a ratty sweater a waitress who's definitely gone through some kinda war with hair all sweaty and dripping across her forehead and smudged and with a pile of greasy dishes in her hands drooling down her sweater and thick glasses yellowed by heat or age and a weary face but smack in the middle of which is the greatest jaw-creaking smile ya ever witnessed and she shows us a table fulla bread crumbs and stained wineglasses and we half-crawl over a business couple to get into the seats and the meal is great original home cooked with no trimmings or fanciness and bowls of steaming veggies carrots all huge poking out from under hot cabbage and a bone and pieces of beef and turnips and with all that there's wine and bread and yogurt and cheese and Jean-Pierre alternates between explaining the dishes to me and talking to the couple at the next table who are interested in us and what we order and we talk about surrealism and certain modern arts and when the meal is over we head back to his place and get down on the tiny cot, this time he's taken it off the springs 'cause the neighbors downstairs suffer when ten consecutive movements are executed on the thing and anyway it's late and we undress and fall into the mattress and make a cool and at the same time frantic love and he shows me afterwards a copy of *The Yage Letters* in French, which I had told him about. He says that he's almost done reading it and he says that he feels very different from Burroughs 'cause Burroughs always has this need to go into bed with young boys and I laugh about that 'cause I realize that my attraction to Burroughs is based on a great deal of his personal mystique, that which has been built up around him by biography and accounts of Burroughsian madness in old letters and magazines and descriptions and the culminating sense of wild head drug stuff that I get off on for the satisfaction of knowing and learning of scenes that connect with maybe unexplored desired areas of sociological truths that are clearly spoken in some of his books and so the letters fell into a perspective that didn't really take heavily the yak about young red-gummed Indians that he wanted to make it with . . . it kinda fell into place with adventure in a mythological and extremely interesting country. And we fell asleep in each other's arms with the window blowing cool winter air into the room and the sleep was strongly horrible with the jumps and turns of bodies on small mattress . . . we woke several times each during the night and in the morning after six hours of half sleep we rose at seven and he sat on the edge of the mattress whispering into my ear and nibbling and smooch in my throat and I asked him if he had difficulty sleeping and he said, Yeah but I understand it is because we are not used to sleeping together and the bed is small and much later he sheepishly said that it was the first time in a year or years that anyone has slept with him overnight in that room . . . he jumped up and so did I hustling on our clothes and rubbing each other's backs and shoulders and warming up to the day . . . the first light of dawn creeping over the roofs and behind the heavy gray curtain of imminent rain.

He took from the window ledge over the courtyard six flights up from the street a tiny package with butter and a half stick of this French bread loaf and we spread butter over it and drank coffee heated from a small stove or hot plate and it tasted like food from the banquets of Monarchs but EVEN BETTER! I loved him madly for a moment where that sense wells up under your throat and spreads like liquor through the system—uhah! We got our stuff together and split from the house in the dawning streets and hustled past the early walkers . . . few out at that hour . . . swept into the car and rode the streets toward the St. George district to pick up my things patting each other on the knees and bellies and all excited about the country common to the senses . . . fall leaves skittering the streets in tiny tornadoes and drifts and turns and posters flapping and a car or two rumbling over the cobblestones and really it's that time of the morning where everything has that fictional sense of otherworldliness and foreign scope of noninhabitation . . . the world's woes wrapped on the edge of night waiting to be freed by movements in the street of the general population and a strong sun that'll illuminate it all to the eye of head and mind. He waited in a café down the block from the rue Laferrière apartment while I went up and downed a couple of cups of hot coffee and brushed my teeth and ate a couple slices of bread and snatched up some clothes and necessities for the trip, journals, etc. I talked with Pat for a little while, a necessary talk concerning some personal stuff she needed to reflect on and then rushed out of the house and into the waiting auto and we were off. We stopped somewhere outside of Paris for gas and then for coffee and small rolls for energy and continued on . . . transcription of the resulting conversations from the ride is almost impossible 'cause of their drift from regular conversations I grapple with in America trying to convey a thought or series of spontaneous senses—and then trying to translate what is not known or understood in the two languages and then there're the word–flights and tangents one goes on to describe the sense of a word . . . damn just sittin' here typetakkin' with two fingers in a flush and rush to get it all down before I fall across these fuckin' keys to bemoan the fact that I'm an open vessel right now of all the erotic and natural sensations and babblings and pulls to the unknown . . . a frightful and exhilarating sense where all is bared and I come face to face on common ground with a sense of my own spirit and life and man there is absolutely no avoiding it . . . it looks ya in the eye and puts a firm hand on your shoulder and says, Kid, this is it . . . continue and step headlong into chance . . . shit . . . the chance to love so entirely that you merge in some sense with another head and yet that chance of being open to another knock in the head and heart if it falls through . . . even in the end you know that it's the gesture, that gesture towards loving that is the most important in the stream of life and consciousness and body and grace . . . So we're rolling along talking about the countryside which is beginning to emerge between desolate factories and civilizscapes and suburbs and now it's rolling hills of dead blond wheat and cows and sheep and moomoo animals and huge fuckin' blackbirds which give a quick example of one section of words from our mouths: He says, Ah see that bird, I like them what are they called in English? Oh uh blackbird or uh magpie . . . Eh? Black baird? Oui oui mugpie? . . . Non, *mag*-pie, like *mag* in *magazine* and *pie,* you know, like grand tart, *pie* . . . Oh oui, oui, well, magpie, ah! Megpie. Ah oui oui . . . You know those birds have special meanings surrounding them, yeah, in English they are considered thieves, voleurs, they fly in your window and steal anything shiny—rings, coins . . . Oh oui? Oui. Ah yes, voleurs, yes, same in French . . . Ah yeah? Yeah, they are my favorite birds, like Edgar Allan Poe ravens . . . Yeah similar to ravens . . . Corneille also in French . . . corn-kneel? Oui oui . . . un blackbaird . . . yeah . . . un l'oiseaux noir. Ah hmm . . . ah . . . oui oui And by this time the bird of the discussion is ten or fifteen kilometers behind us and winging off in directions of the wind and we point out other discoveries in the landscape, cows take on added pleasurable meanings and little goats and baby oinkers and the trees of soft gold floating effortlessly in the foggy distance and soon the sun has broken through the mist and I say, Yeah, a symbol, two seconds later it gets dark again with fog . . . secretly embarrassed at this knock at my pleasurable symbol . . . silly notions circling my mind . . . He takes my hand at times and lifts it to his mouth and sucks on my forefinger and tongues it wet chills into the palm of my hand and I'm half delirious and every time we're stuck behind a slow car on a long curved stretch, I mutter, Escargots . . . he giggles and says, Oui oui, and at times I reach over and caress his belly under his warm sweater and chills run through my spine and heart and my hands sweat at the palms and every so often he leans over and kisses me on the lips and I'm amazed as if it's never happened before like this . . . and I drift in thoughts like great collages of senses and past images of the previous evening and projected scenes of later and I get hot in the forehead almost like fever and in the midst of all this at the end or near end of the three-hour drive I get struck by this sense like some great revealing section of his mind and body has suddenly merged within my bloodstream and I'm breathing a sense of him in such a way that we are just about indistinguishable, this is all in silence in the car with landscape drifting and what I suddenly feel is that he is mine and in some sense possessed within my coarsing blood in my pores, not a selfish owning sense but just a total merge within and at that exact moment in comes arrowlike a realization that he is an entirely separate person and living independent of me and my blood and that it's a subtle unknown thing that has drawn us together that is by no means certain or everlasting and from that I feel a striking and sudden faintness, a fever in my throat and forehead and my hands tremble invisibly and I'm about to black out in this fever and wanna grab onto something for all the frightening bareness I feel like a solitary kid drifting through all this time and space and landscape searching for connection and a vast unexplainable feeling that has a tag called love . . . it's all here in front of me and I have fears of it ending at some indeterminable point in some future and yet feel that this has taken place as it's meant to be and whatever comes of it, continuance or ending at any time, it still has to be felt in the blood 'cause in that I have no choice . . . we arrive home in Hauteville la fuichard and stop in Mesnil la vigot grocery and gas station for supplies and rush on home and light a fire and there's letters waiting from Janine Vega/ Charlie Plymell/Alex Rodriguez/Harold Biddle . . . the letters are beautiful so fuckin' great they warm an already warmed heart and Alex makes me wanna cry for the New York scenes and Charlie thrills me with his genuine talk of my manuscript having shown it to Anne Waldman and in the process of putting me in contact with German publishers for maybe my prose and he seems to enjoy my letters and look forward to 'em and then Janine with her fuckin' beautiful heart-talk of her life and sense of it and things that correlate to things I feel and don't articulate and a great poem and talk of Dennis and his lover and good commonheart sense and Harold dear Harold with his sensitive eye and heart and need for contact like all of us saying he might now go to hairdressing school 'cause bookies closed up and he's working on stories to send out to mags having not written too much before and I'm glad things have taken on perspective for him . . . he's going to school for high school diploma and it's weary-sad but I love him for his senses . . .

I let Jean-Pierre read Janine's letter he gets stuck on the slang and purposefully misspelled words, which I try to explain to him as an earthy quality and a communication removed from the bourgeois social structure, language of the street and the working class, language of the heart moving out to communicate with someone in the distance . . . he has difficulty understanding the letter anyway and gives up on it after a page but that's okay 'cause someday I'll speak français well enough to translate for him the deliriously beautiful content of these messages across the waters . . . we take a tumble on the couch and get sweaty but break it off for a long walk before sunset to the soccer field scene of glorious desperate fantasies and down into the town past the three guerrillas on the hillside rusted and popping in the elements past the gas station where the ragged little mutt yaps and squeals at us and further down around the church of that town to where a bridge crosses a stream and in the distance is green green long grass fields . . . Jean-Pierre says, Valleys, and Yes it is . . . with great forlorn cows dotting the lines of hills and meadows and small tucked farmhouses and low rolling traces of mist and sun breaking through clouds illuminating like the colored plates of magic books and we turn to this fenced-in area by the bridge with a very weary watchdog who calmly walks over to the fence, just doing my duty folks never you pay me no mind but don't be foolish enough to try and take my fish 'cause he's guarding a trout breeding pool where there's incredible high leaps of fish into the air and underwater scurrying movement of the whole load of them fighting for drifting insects and we walk all the way back up the long steep hill tossing a green apple back and forth in leaps and bounds . . .

We stopped on the road to ask the price of fresh-killed chicken and agreed to return and buy one in an hour after the farmer's wife kills and cleans it for us and we head home to clean veggies and drink coffee and talk and I try to explain my manuscript to him, my life and senses in a series of words and scenes and contacts and interests that takes very little time and is compact full of truths and revelations and for that I am glad for wherever this goes it will at least go openhearted . . .

We rush out after two hours of lolling around and talking and realize we're late for the blasted chicken and we roll down the road the air so damn crisp it frosts the windows and freezes the vision and we're alternately wiping and rubbing the windows and making turns and swerves and yeah the chicken is ready for us we yaktak with the farmer his wife and beautiful clear-eyed kids at the kitchen table and ride back and the chicken's popped into the oven and later when it's done all brown and roasted in cloves of garlic and carrots and potatoes and onions and my mouth drops at this incredible meal Jean-Pierre has come up with and we eat humming and umming and ah yeah oui oui great slurp and a li'l wine to freshen the spirit

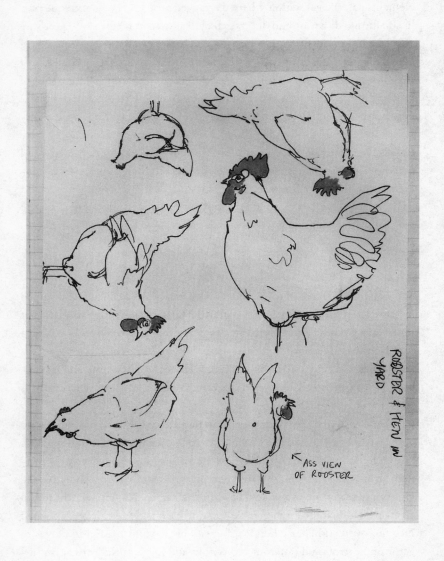

ROOSTER & HEN IN YARD

ASS VIEW OF ROOSTER

and cheese and yogurt for dessert and after that we talk about bats and owls and get into bed . . . so fuckin' cold without the heater working that the skin almost freezes to the sheets . . . he undresses quick and ouch ouch jumps beneath the sheets moaning at the freeze of them and I undress and . . . ah . . . ah . . . inch my way beneath the covers and we rub and warm each other up breathing hot breath on each other's bodies to chase the chill away and soon that becomes frenzy and we're getting on in the heat of delicious sexual contact the sheets go flying off it doesn't matter anymore the heat has come up from the heart into the surface of flesh and eyes glowing we roll back and forth and finally there is sleep . . . long restful uninterrupted smooth warm exterior interior sleep where dreams chase the hedges and dogs wheel around the sky and not a river or snake or any sexual image but the strongest one of all and its rhythms of life itself ah yeah . . .

Wake up this morning with him kissing my throat and ears and nibbling on my lobes and breathing warm sounds in me like life into deflated heart and it's rosy-colored sky breaking in the windows and sun soon to come around to us and coffee gets put on the stove . . . a hustle into warm clothes and an attack in the direction of breakfast: ham sliced up and eggs laid out over the ham till there's a delicious crispy edge to 'em and hot eye-jolting coffee and kisses across the table and we get into the car to go to the sea, chickens running about clucking crazily and we ride off windows open smoking on cigarettes and getting lost at times backtracking and finding the right directions and finally after a long ride around we get to the sea, not the same areas as I've been to before but a new one further up the coast and it's beautiful we're the only ones there in sight surrounded by huge cliff-dunes and the sandy shore curves like a serpent around for a few miles . . . we dodge the tides sinking in sand at spots leaping over mysterious rivulets and collecting interesting rocks. I'm looking for white rocks and smooth ones for rock paintings and he brings me some every now and then and at one point has to take a wicked piss so he says it's poetic pissing in the ocean . . . I say yeah it's a defiant confrontation between man and nature . . . watch the tide will roll away when he pisses, retreating he whizzes into the ocean and I think he looks beautiful he comes towards me and takes me in his arms and we kiss silent long and slowly lingering on the tips of tongues and the warm wind from a hidden sun behind the gauze of thin clouds comes bristling our hairlines and I remember earlier there was a phone call to his parents and he has to return to Paris this evening or early early tomorrow morning and I suddenly miss him already as I'm standing there in his arms with my mouth against his throat . . . with the jagged tip of a broken shell I draw Aztecian turtles and serpents and crabs and phallic shapes and he makes comments on each one according to a language composed of a series of delighted grunts and ahs and ums and we return slowly to the car after an hour of sea breeze and ride slowly home through tiny towns with smiling families and kids in French yards playing solitary games of mythological importance with themselves and great rosy handsome faces from toil and sea air and flashes of shell white teeth and we're at the turn into Mesnil la vigot having come from a different direction and there we stop again at the gas station grocery for some veggies and fruit and we head home where he transforms the chicken from last night into a great hearty stew with fresh salad and he says he relaxes when he's cooking so enjoys it and that's evident when ya sink your mouth into a forkful of this stuff juices brimming to the edge of your tongue . . . in the wait before it was finished he came out and sat and watched me drawing a thick serpent in India ink and water-colors on the most perfect stone in the enormous shirtful I dragged back with me about twenty-five stones and this one was round and smooth and the serpent on it was coiling in squirmy thrusts and with colors of a sad rainbow that'll never be shown in the sky in my lifetime . . . one area a color where I painted a thin glaze of orange around the bright red spots and then coated the orange with a thin thin layer of indigo blue so a strange and remote color like the color of the desert in its final angle came up and the bright red spots of the markings of the snake within this color were enough to make the snake wriggle right off the stone and I sprayed it with shellac and called him over to the open doorway where the sun shone strongest and showed him the finished piece which he liked a lot and then told him it was for him for a souvenir of the last two days and he smiled embarrassedly and kissed me quickly and we sat down with coffee and I told him how strange it was in the house with him because the three weeks I had spent alone I had fantasized what it'd be like to have a person with me there, a

warm body to sleep with and warm heart to communicate with . . . I realized when we first arrived how the whole fuckin' house was stretched and
hung with an enormous load of fantasy from my periods of solitude—whole
images colliding in the corners of the ceiling and windows and along the
grass fields outside and so I was nervous which I didn't convey to him but
I think was transmitted subtly in the jerks of my hands and legs and now
there was a warm fire in the fireplace and we made love on the couch and
afterwards ate dinner in the kitchen talking about so many things and my
French had actually improved so much over the last two days I was speaking sentences to him with occasional English thrown in when I didn't know
a word. We talked about Eastern religion and I told him I didn't know much
about it but had I ever the desire to get into such a thing it would indeed be
some form of Eastern religion as Western ones were too prostituted and
controlled and distorted by papal and clerical creeps and it was interesting
what came from the conversation as he was surprised I realized certain things
about the spirit and the vibrations of the spirit in all things animate and
inanimate and there came that point where he had to leave and I kissed him
long and slow and he left in the night out in his car me standing in the porch
below the incredible freeze of stars in the sky the clearest night in a long
time and the semifrozen moon bright and clear no bats wheeling around
too cold for 'em and he finally backed the car out and turned waved and
rolled out onto the road and I came inside and put on some music and made
some coffee and sat down at the typewriter to record all this not just for
posterity's sake but to fight off the woeful sense of his leaving which hits
hard in the chest and the head and to keep myself doing something so I
don't sink and because it's so cold in the house I'm feeling it suddenly more
so now that he's gone and silence has invaded every corner and the past
days have been drifting in through my head down to my feet each little
moment of illumination of what he is to me suddenly coming clear and sharp
and I finally broke down wailing over these fucking keys 'cause I have
reached that sense where I feel a strength suddenly alive in this ol' heart of
mine so new and strong and here to stay that relief brought it all out in sa-
line water and I'm afraid to get into bed with all the senses it now holds and
before he left in the silence of the dinner table he said he felt funny about

leaving so soon and I tried to make him feel better by pretending it was completely understandable and that he had to go and it's been really nice that he was able to be here the last two days and then as he sat there in silence he suddenly said, Well I think of how difficult it is for you not to be able to speak to anyone around here . . . I said, Yeah, in the three weeks I was here alone I only spoke seven times, four times to people and three times to myself, just to hear the vocal cords buzz after an incredible period of silence where the body calms in such a way as to make you aware of sounds you never noticed before, sounds and rhythms of the woods and trees and unseen animals day and night and the hum of the ground in walking and that for those reasons I had to occasionally break the silence and exercise my own audible form of communication and he nodded in agreement and now it's late night and there is a silence composed of both the night and the absence of a fellow that I have somehow connected with so's to feel the emergence of a viable sense in my blood and bones and all I can do is lay down and rest this head and gather energy in the sleep of things and understand it all in such a way as to feel the thanks for it regardless of any outcome . . . and I still have the sense of him around me the taste of his flesh on my tongue among the sheets among the cool interiors of the house and the moon develops a thin haze around its shell curve and riding to the sea this afternoon I repeated slowly the sections of his body and mind that sent chills through my system until everything was covered, his face cheeks the flat rippled stomach the legs the mind the slow utterance of words the ideas that surface in loose talk the arms and thin wrists and the taste of him and the awarenesses of things going on the warmth of his brown eyes the crow black hair tattering down the sides of his neck the warm spot in the wells of his shoulders the feet and the toes and the chest and the teeth and the warm breath that tickles my sides and neck and the forehead which holds so much and the explanation he gave me of having majored in philosophy in school and how it means nothing in terms of the walking working world and I laughed and said a friend in New York took philosophy and someone once asked him what he would do with it after school was over and he said, Drive a cab . . . and falling into the cold cold bed alone I realized how quickly it would have been warm had he been there to touch me and talking aloud to myself to calm my senses the words coming slow from my lips saying: my hands my arms my thoughts and all I can do is write yes that's all I could do . . .

After I tried to stuff the subject when he said he felt funny about leaving so soon, me pretending that it was all understandable (it was) and that that's the way things go (really I felt sad to see him go) and there was a look in his eyes that made me feel it'd be best to put my heart on my sleeve and not pretend it wasn't affecting me so I said, Ya know . . . I feel . . . and I couldn't articulate it so I stopped, he turns and looks up and says, Yes? What do you feel? . . . I said, Ah, never mind it's nothing . . . He said, Tell me what do you feel, do you feel cold? Ah no, I said, It ain't that . . . well it's just that I really enjoyed you being here for the last two days . . . it was really good, ya know?

December 11, 1978

Jean-Pierre and I went to the sea again, this time in an area I am familiar with, the ride slow and beautiful weaving in among stone towns and high walls and labyrinth roads and coasting through tunnels of trees in the approach to the rise overlooking the sea—time measureless as usual in situations where all my concern lies within a palm on my knee or softly caressing the belly and it was getting on towards evening cigarettes dangling from the corners of our mouths and slow-motion coasting up the hilly road with dark shadows spreading out over the roads from the trees and we pull over onto the bristly grass dunes and walk down to the sea . . . shades of Fellini with young painted-face girls in blooming fur coats walking with a waggle of the hips down the sand past old weathered fishermen and couples sleeping curled in the sand before their incredibly long poles stuck down into the beach with lines trailing into invisibility in the surf . . . the water a very strange blue ratty dogs barking from different spots at us . . . the sky turns pale blue rosy and the sun forms into a flowering ball with fissures of flame and colorless jets streak pounding the air and after collecting some stones for me and walking the surf we head back to the car right around the time the sun disappears and ride back out through the tree-lined road and through

the towns and up around hills and stretches of asphalt in the gathering light
. . . I have his cock out of his pants and stimulating him in a crazy scene and
it's getting intense we roll down a hill past a cop van with whirling blue
light and we turn into the road that leads to Hauteville la guichard and it's
pure night blooming along the thick spread of trees and scraggly bushes and
we pull over to the side of the road the erotic sense too strong to continue
and lock into a deep wet kiss and bodies thrusting and my pants find their
way down to my ankles his tongue tracing cool wet curves over my throat
and neck and shoulder-wells and down to my belly and my hands are wet
with saliva and caressing his cock and rubbing his chest and my eyes half-
closed with passion from his face and skin I see the mosaic trees emitting
soft blue steely glints of rapid night last light sky and white spots of black
cows moving glacierlike behind the trees and the gullies shuddering patches
of blue-black and sounds of crickets and night birds looming among the
trees and he's down near my ankles kissing slow trails up my legs over onto
my hands and back to my sides and over my cock the unbelievably warm
sense of his mouth over my cock up and down and brush of lips and up to
my throat again and I repeat the actions for his pleasure and his stomach is
hard as a rock thrusting under my palms and lips passion as an elevator in
the shape of red lights rising beneath the steel surface as a needle thrust into
veins canalling the arms and legs and throbbing temples pulse, like the heat
of nests and bellies of birthing creatures and needles of night shooting from
surfaces of unseen things into red ruby eyes, as the taillights of this coasting
vehicle having come to a final stop among the trees rolling over dead leaves
burst of color behind my eyes and breathing becoming fog-dense and uttered sounds slick as stream stones and algae tongue coasting down the valleys and structure of flesh in a movement of frenzied life before the advancing
wall of flame, of forest fires and aging and dreams having uttered before the
plains distance of the eyes and the heart, coasting machines of complex media-
flash and smiling assholes winking from the doors of brand-new Cadillacs
and smoking brand-name cigarettes an ad like on highway billboards and
all that drifts down in my skull with wind rising and consuming this solitary
vehicle in the rasp of forestry and lonesomeness of men and the desires the
world sees behind the soft spots of its knees so suddenly that the reaction is

to blot out and deny but the world can go fuck itself as far as "humanity" and "need for law": outlaws drift in every vehicle of thought coming down this hillside—cars ride way down the valleys of sunsets and gathering night where the world is laid out in dark shadows of color behind and in front of the windshield in the ruts that line the roads and the gullies that attempt to climb from their places of the earth and extend themselves to the sky and reach the dying sun before chance comes in the morning to claim their movements and momentary freedoms and send them splashing back down into places all outlined and set within the manmade history of things . . .

CONCERNING REPETITIONS IN MY WRITING! "REAL THINKING IS CONCEPTIONS AIMING AGAIN AND AGAIN AND ALWAYS GETTING FULLER, THAT IS THE DIFFERENCE BETWEEN CREATIVE THINKING AND THEORISING." — GERTRUDE STEIN

Wild Horses

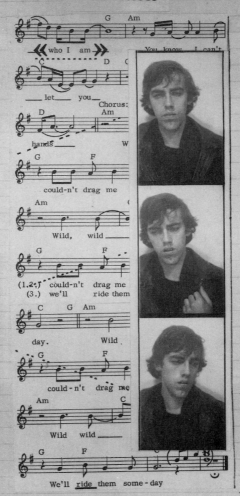

who I am   You know   I can't

___ let ___ you ___

hands ___   W

could-n't drag me

Wild,   wild ___

(1.2.) could-n't   drag me
(3.) we'll   ride them

day.   Wild

could-n't   drag me

Wild   wild ___

We'll ride them some-day

the horse is galloping off into the russet dusk of the seas — VISION IS LESS
elastic —

December 2, 1978

Sent off manuscript to Sylvia. Cost me 7F, which I really could not afford. Felt like shit afterwards as she laid it out pretty clearly that she had no intention of using it, maybe just for *Gasolin 23* but otherwise no dice. Shouldn't have given it to her, putting myself in a position for semistarvation. That fucking 7F coulda bought three cans of soup or a package of chicken or a huge piece of Gruyère or two chocolate bars or stamps and envelopes or six yogurts or two packs Gauloises filtres or . . .

December 3, 1978

Walked among the tomb-silent buildings, marble structures pushing up from the ground with glass squares nodding sections of airless winter sky, rusty cans and newspapers drifted across dirt lots and the surfaces of walkways, a feeling of nausea at the soundlessness of things, at hands surging from the ends of my coat sleeves. I realized for a moment what madness is or can come from—the unstable relation of the body with the environment, a sense like a knife poised forever a centimeter away from the wet surface of your eye, a sadness mixing with all that. At the lines engraving themselves into my forehead and palms, a time of aging when I feel I have not yet arrived at the unmarked X of my desires, the vortex of senses in relation to the world that always, elusive and indefinable, waits beyond, around the corner. I had a strange vision, don't know how or why, whether it was a product of the moment or a culmination of the threads of physical chance, turning a concrete angle of the overlapping walkways I saw up on a dirt mound high above the leveling of the field a bristly piglike animal scratching at the earth,

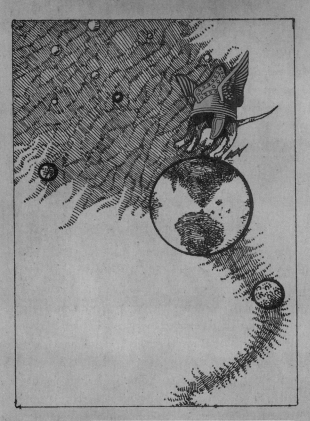

a dream touches down upon the earth
in the night...

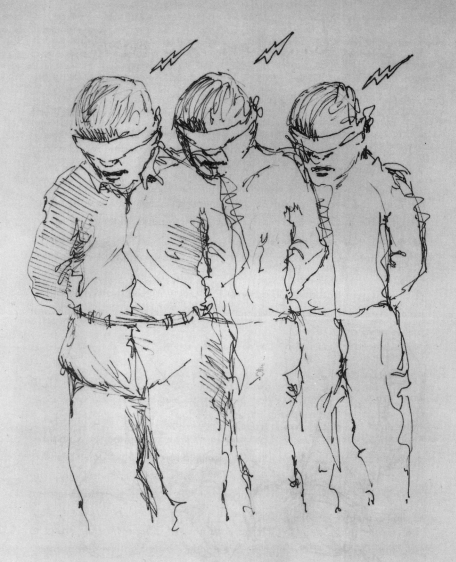

Trembling figure before firing squad.
                        Paris 1.15.78

(after Duchamp)

pummeling it with its fore and hind paws, raising clouds of dry dust which immediately disappeared in contact with the slight and sudden rain. But somehow it seemed right. After all, here I was in the center of Paris, in the center of life itself, my life, a foreign animal who seemed not to belong anywhere anymore: the irises, retinas, the spherical orbiting balls in this head seeing everything now from a strange and unimaginable distance, like the distances of the forest in the eyes of the fish, in the sea swirling round within the thick blue heart of the horse. I wanted to embrace that hyena, that spotted bristled pig, lay down and pummel the earth alongside it, looking for the door, the door that leads away, the entrance into some semblance of recognizable and believable environment, something soothing for this weary heart, this weary head, something that would enable the two of us, foreign brothers in blood, brains, and sight, to lay back drifting, drifting on a huge and warm vellum of polar ice, in the Ferris wheel of night and do nothing else but stay up and trade blood with the stars, with the showering tails of lonely comets while a fragrant blue veil of life drifts through the night and makes us its own.

December 4, 1978

Picked up my certificate of attendance from Alliance Français with Jean-Pierre this morning. We went on to the police station up behind Blvd. St.-Germain/Notre-Dame. They will send me an appointment within three weeks to get my Cuit de ses jours. We walked through St.-Michel together stopping at a German bakery for a cheese/raisin Danish pie and I split from there at the Odéon metro to return to St. George and the rue Laferrière apartment. Worked a bit more on Jimmy Romano's tape, been playing with the circuits of the radio which has a number of different bands, brings in England very well. Been doing a cut-up experiment with different music and English talk shows, also with the electronic frequencies that come through at different points on the dial. Some unbelievable words trapped on the tape, a section of a talk show on terrorists in which some pig "explained" the sexual thrill women get from armed revolution. Couldn't believe the woman heading the show, who sounded slightly progressive, would let him get away with that. I'd have slapped him rightly across the kisser. Am feeling a bit nervous concerning this afternoon's meeting with Nidra Poller, wondering what's gonna come of it all, in regards to my working here in Paris and also in regards to the manuscript. Christ, I wanna have the thing published bad. It's important to me in a number of ways. I guess acceptance is one of them, the publishing of it being symbolic acceptance of the importance of it, that which I feel is evident. When I get my typewriter, a job, an apartment, I wanna work on a new manuscript of my semisurreal writings and send it to C.B. [Christian Bourgois].

6:10 P.M. Just got back from meeting Nidra Poller. Showed up at her apartment and was met at the door by a fella, I asked for Nidra and she came out of a room nearby. A fairly short woman with beautiful frizzy brown hair, intense knowledgeable eyes, she's somewhere in her thirties. She invited me into a room stacked with great books—American and French publishers. We talked for a while, she didn't know of any prospects for work but that didn't matter so much after I talked with her more. She explained her interest in the manuscript as she had not too long ago finished a big novel constructed entirely of voices: two characters holding the arena for whatever length of time they walk and then replaced with two other characters. She tried to remove herself as much from the act of writing as was possible, thus the characters were not as well written as she would have liked but they had much to say. Much freedom in that. The manuscript was read by senior editors in a load of publishers in America but all said it wasn't something they could sell. Recently another woman wrote a book in France that was all voices and was received with much ado: "First time in literature," etc. She asked me what I drew as a conclusion from the manuscript I wrote and I said, I didn't conclude anything, that it was an act to place outside myself the responsibility of having been the receiver of the related tales, that it was an uncomfortable feeling being in contact with family and friends and having that knowledge of events taking place in faceless characters' lives, that no one with stability or routine would ever have the chance to meet these characters. She said she was happy with her stability and so

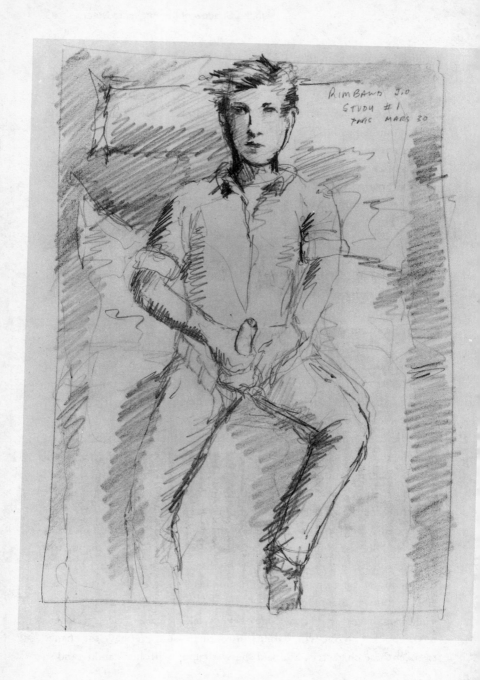

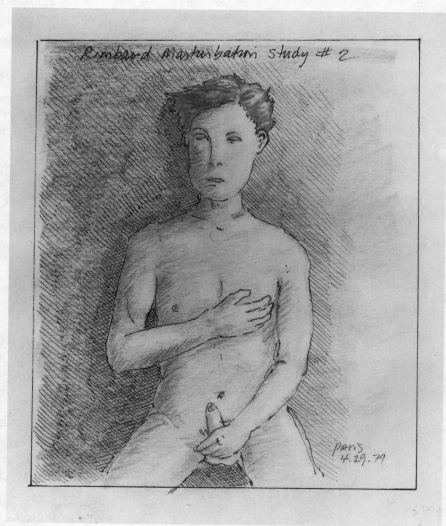

Rimbaud Masturbation study # 2

paris
4.29.79

would never be in the position to meet these characters, thus an added interest in the book. She served me coffee and let me check out a copy of *WOZU*[?], an anthology of writings just out from Soleil Noir. It looked pretty impressive, one poem in it by Ferlinghetti which surprised me, it was very good and connected with a lot of my senses of searching in life and writing, surprised me as I haven't felt too much for his writings in a while, his later stuff being to me more repetitious word output. She talked about a novel she was wanting to write about the relationship between mother and daughter. Sounded like a fantastic piece the way she described it, saying that she was waiting for her position to change so as to start, that she did not want to write it out of anxiety or nervous energy or any sense that would come from a definite approach. She talked of developing her erotic writings, that nothing she has read has ever appealed to her erotic senses. She wanted to get away from seeing characters in writing from a distance, getting close up in order to write the erotic senses of the "intelligent body," the "thinking body," not the usual body separated from mind. We talked about much more, which I won't bother to relate here as it was about senses I received in the course of conversation that hit well and hard in connection with me. I leave all that inside me—also have to rush off to class at Alliance Français.

I GOT LIVIN' ON MY SIDE
(lyrics—work in progress)

I got livin' on my side
but it don't buy me a place to sleep
not a place to lay my body (head)
don't buy me food to eat

it don't buy me no wheels
it don't buy me ma pills
it don't buy me heaven
it only buy me hell
it only buy me hell

it don't buy me no meals
only what I go out and steal
unless I go on out and steal
whatever I go out and steal

dreams come fast in the summertime
but baby it's goin' on winter soon
I broke as a hanged bandit

like kickin' a rock in the river
it ain't ever comin' back no more

got living on my side
but it don't buy me a set a wheels
don't buy me my pills
only what I go out and steal

oh time   time   time   got your shoulder
leaving me nothin' to cry on

I got livin' on my side
but it don't gimme someone to lie on

it's so easy with whiskey whiskey
so easy with amphetameenze
my rooms so cheap it ain't got windows
makes it hard to figure out my dreams

in the town square they talk like dogs
up in the offices they grunt like hogs
it never really is what ya figure it'll be
unless ya figure out the drunken key
unless ya got a copy of the sideshow key

March 18–June 1, 1979
New York or Ocean
Journal de L'Homme Ordinaire—
Journal of the Ordinary Man

April 11, 1979 (Wednesday)

Looking through this sparse journal dated from mars 18, I see so little in the way of internal mapping. Most is external as usual in all the journals, the internal is stuff that isn't threatening/embarrassing. Well, have to stop this, the words *cryptic* and *symbolist* on page 16 of this journal were referring to my meeting a young Englishman my own age in the jardin des Tuileries. What was extremely funny (not in hilarious sense but in amusing coincidental realizations) was that this mirrored my last days in New York before arriving here. I brought the fellow home and we made love and afterwards talked about getting together again, he suggesting that I come for dinner on Tuesday the tenth. In lying together among the tangled sheets we talked while I smoked a cigarette and dreamed towards the white ceiling watching the smoke whirl through the sunlight. I felt somewhat relieved in going to bed with another person other than Jean-Pierre especially in light of the fact I am leaving, it was sort of a removal point, difficult to deal with my leaving him and also there was some sort of breakthrough in lying down with a boy of my own age. Most of my growing up since my first sexual experience with a man has been in the arms of older men, men in their thirties and forties, not so much that I desire older men for age but for their grasp on life, the settling down inside of themselves, some kind of calm and reassurance and proof of life; dunno how to make this clear as I've never pondered it much except in odd moments and now as I grow older I desire younger and younger men though I don't usually sleep with anyone younger than me and rarely someone my own age or even close mostly because of their awkwardness and my desire to relate to someone who has a lot more thinking and reflecting behind him. It also occurred to me that possibly I have always slept with older men because of some kind of inherent security, that the age difference separates me from them to an extent, thereby giving me a sense that I can say what I want and if it's not accepted by them I can always attribute this to their position in time and aging; this is not to be unfair to myself, it's just a slight possibility and I don't know if it is invented or real. There is something a bit frightening to me about relationships with someone my own age in way of lovemaking, etc., but now with this Englishman I felt relieved of any thoughts concerning the whole subject; it no longer exists with the intensity it once did. I even felt an infatuation with him after he left, similar to meeting Phillip while involved with Randy, with Phillip it drove me against the wall that I was leaving after meeting such a down-to-earth guy, him and his childhood Stetson camping out in the rolling hills of Montana . . . that kind of suburban innocence hmm . . . so the problem was in explaining to Jean-Pierre that I wanted to go to dinner and possibly we would have sex, me and this English guy (Alan). It took several days to work up to the subject; in the meantime I was alternating between feelings of possibly being very wrong considering that I was involved with J.P. for this long and that it might hurt him if I was to do so. Then came senses of myself as a human being who needed freedom to do exactly what he desired in way of contact, sexual or otherwise . . . I always am consumed in this sense that I should be able to move where and when I desire; I wouldn't give up my relationship with J.P. for another person in the way of commitment, just need to explore things as they move my way . . . images of floating from room to room and bed to bed and country to country and time to time . . . just moving as chance brings me and at the same time being involved with one person who I feel comfortable with for a period of time, someone I can relax and be myself, allow any thoughts changes, etc., to come forth.

Okay I told Jean-Pierre and he said, You must feel free to do as you wish.

Fine, now days later last night I left for Alan's house and stopped by J.P.'s job to give him the keys to the apartment and standing there I asked him if he truly understood, I was worried he might not, that I did love him and yet this was necessary. He said, This isn't the time to talk about it. I left through the driving rain and caught a metro to St. Lazare station and found Alan's house after much walking around and searching streets for the right avenue. He lives upstairs on the seventh floor of an old building with court-yard, student sorts of rooms, creaking staircases and dank hallways and drip-ping pipes, recalling the roach havens I lived in on the Lower East Side near Bowery mission—whines and howls of babies and dogs. Heard the sound of a radio program from the BBC down the dark hallways and followed it to his door, he was bent over with a pair of red rubber gloves on, cuttin' up celery and apples for our meal. I went inside and he struggled with one glove, pulled it off and extended his hand for a shake. I sat down in the room at the table, a wobbly chair. It was a small room, very small with old crumb-littered rug disappearing beneath a tiny cot, the roof/ceiling sloped down at a sharp angle and a tiny skylight with one broken pane opened out so that if you stood up your head would go through and peer out over rainy gray Paris roofs. A nudie calendar with some Swedish blonde woman with taut nipples breasts and sitting against a cheesy backdrop was on one wall, chestnut branches in bloom pushing from an old juice bottle filled with scummy green water and a sink that didn't work. We listened to the news for a half hour while he cut the vegetables and fruit and poured out nuts over them; vegetarian he is. Okay so during dinner we talked of mundane things, somehow just no click of personalities, I realized my infatuation and then the senses slid away. He's an amiable guy, seems to know a lot more about American media culture than I do, which is okay granted I never watch the tube at home and don't really care a bit for any of it. He told me of this girl he knew: She was born of a rich family who were all communists, her brothers became lawyers and defended many students during the May Day clash aftermath, she became a nun and after some time realized that wasn't quite what she needed in her life, her parents died and left her a château in the south of France, she created a triangle between France America and some other country, riding about on jets and fucking everywhere, she liked to be tied into chairs and roughed up a bit not beaten badly but slight sadism, more the desire for the threat of it following with wild lovemaking than the actual beatings. She soon created the triangle involving Canada rather than the States as she had met an American who beat her quite badly, I asked her, Why Canada I mean I thought you went in for roughhousing. She replied, Those Americans are too bloody literal. Now she has retired to the château and raises a large garden. I went to her house; her family was always a bit eccentric and didn't go in for furniture of any sort, so in going to her château one must sit on the floor, eat on the floor, and watch television on the floor, no rugs or such so that these enormous slugs would go trailing their slime all over the floors of the house, she would say, Oh my, look at that one, aren't they marvelous creatures?

At one point I wanted to leave quite badly, the place was great but I was feeling slightly claustrophobic for as we got into bed it was so extremely small that I could not move an inch without falling out. Rain tapping on my head through the broken skylight and some alley or roof cat yowling away like a banshee out in the night . . . We made love and talked in the dark, I tried fucking him but he had difficulty in doing so, so we masturbated together. Of course in all this time I did not forget J.P. in fact I thought of him each hour, each hour wishing I hadn't said I'd spend the night, wanting to rise up put on my jeans and split and head home through the dark streets and take a shower and climb into bed with Jean. He asked me if I liked threesomes and I said my two experiences with them were awfully awkward and therefore not enjoyable, no way to move naturally among two other bodies, always elbows in the face or knees in the balls, that sort of thing. He suggested possibly he call a friend some other time and all of us get it on. I murmured a noncommittal answer. It's extremely easy to find the reasons for not wanting to be involved with a person; but that sort of thing isn't necessary for me, if I feel uncomfortable by way of a relationship with a guy I simply don't get into it further than it's gone. I realized the extent of my infatuation and fluctuated between feelings of being a fool for not staying home that night, or at least *not* staying the *night* here at Alan's. I still feel he's a nice guy but I am leaving and I do want to spend my time with Jean-Pierre and Brian when he arrives. Besides, what I felt was possible between Alan and me was a good communication with humor and illumination—not so. We are too far apart culturally and in our vision/scope of life itself, he being content to talk about media scenes, me wanting to talk about life. More important, me wanting to learn about my senses more, feel more comfortable with my leanings and travel movements

Woke up at six o'clock and in the gray light got dressed and kissed him good-bye and descended the rattling stairs to the courtyard, through the heavy doors to the street, ogres of concierges leaning over ground-floor sills with puffed alcoholic faces leering toothless grins in my direction as I walked down the street, up in the sky huge black blankets of rolling clouds passing over roofs and in the far east a billowing line of gold breathing light, of sunrise spectacular and life-filled and I hurried home to St. Georges, stopping for a croissant for J.P. and thinking of him being up by now shaving with his customary sink of cold water and hard razor blade, the dog yapping for its breakfast and the look upon opening the door between our eyes, I passed loads of stupid cops as usual in the doorways and streets all peering about with dead glazed eyes for action, went upstairs opened the door, J.P. was nude in the bathroom before the mirror with shaving cream on his face and a line of blood trickling among the white, he's cut himself again, I always tell him to use warm water but we exchanged ça va's and I sat down at the kitchen table with a cup of steaming coffee and sighed. He came out a bit later and sat down acting as if there was nothing happening between us; me filled with all these wondering senses of what he thinks and feels about last night my not returning home. As for the north shore it seems he's no longer going to go for three days but will make it the week and wants to be alone for a few days by himself up there, thus I would return myself by train with the dog. I realize now the change in plans and of course why; needless to reiterate here . . . So I guess I'll stay here alone all week and he can spend all the time at the shore by himself, I resist senses of being made to split at some time for someone else's solitude, though all this time his only vacation aside from August being next week, somehow I feel sensitive to his asking for the time alone meaning away from me. Again it's understood but I would feel better not going at all than to have to pick up my things and take a train back alone . . . I guess it's the move of *having* to leave, *being* the object of intrusion . . . Many things for me to do here, to complete or prepare for leaving, some writings I want to finish, also the call expected from Brian. Again today, all this morning I've thought about J.P. and Brian and past and present relationships and realize I have to stress to any and all persons I become involved with that I must be able to do what I wish, it is my life and my senses and it can be called selfishness, but I absolutely have never been able to put myself in a position where I deny chance and other ways of movement, whether over distances and landscapes or in lovemaking. It's the settling down that is so difficult; choosing one form excludes all others, the only answer is not choosing at all but merely moving under one's own will; this is something that angers many people, that many people find faulty and that many people say is an avoidance of responsibility; maybe so but then again I am alive and I am continually distracted by movements around me and alternative things, continually looking searching for traces of my life and others amongst the landscapes.

The difficulty I have at times is in wondering whether to trust my vision—my image and view of things and why they exist, rationalizations, you might say. I realize the ease with which anyone might find reasons to support whatever viewpoints they hold or to support whatever actions they may wish to make . . . How more or less true or real is this from any alternative way of seeing or believing?

. . . ain't it always a silly mess of senses, really now, all this shoulda been spared from the typewriter . . . I wonder if I'm alive years from now will I appreciate this or scorn the very idea of it . . . this self-searching in the face of a world that kills people with bombs . . .

April 19, 1979

The gray sea dawn silvery like a television screen flickering through the windows at various times in the night and morning. Waking several times on my back and arms uplifting to ward off the night, the morning, the hopelessness of no sleep, the images of closed eyes still running as I return to them, turning over heavily in the sheets: I'm in some suburban town, a New Jersey sense in the air, old houses and colonial-style pillared boxes and most of them white with soft glow among the night trees and lanes, I'm moving through, soft whisper of shapes of people in cars and on foot moving in and out of darkness on their ways home or to bars or to other houses, looking for a bar that's open, seeing the blush of red neon down some tree-swept street and figuring on buying a pack of cigarettes. Somewhere in these scenes, dogs bark and children move along and I meet Syd, the Jersey lawyer who was my second dad during Times Square street routines, met him hustling and we traded our minds bare from then on in various hotels, various states, states of mind, states of distance, he's really grown so much older as I have too, he hands me a couple of letters that he's written to me, I see staples in one, something affixed to the back of the letter, money I imagine . . . I stuff it into my pocket, too embarrassed to read it and look to see what's affixed on its back in front of him. I'm alone and moving through the streets, wind tossing dark trees almost invisible in the perspective of night, in the foyer of some house, I meet Syd's wife, we talk real friendly, though I've never met her before, she's very nice and we talk loose and then I pull something, cigarettes maybe, out of my pocket and when I turn away for a moment and then turn back, she is standing there in the near darkness of the living room unfolding one of the letters Syd gave me, I can see his name and his handwriting and his law firm letterhead on the paper. She recognizes it immediately. I rush over and feel an acute pain in my senses and rip it out of her hands, she turns and looks at me sadly, a bit shocked, not knowing what the letter was, not having time to read it, but knowing it was from her husband to me, I feel terrible and try to explain to her, it's something she wouldn't understand, that it belongs to me, I'm sorry for having to take it away like that. She finds the second letter on the floor, I take that from her with equal force, feeling even worse, she knows something is wrong, still doesn't quite know the exact truth, I feel it's better she doesn't. Syd is on the phone, she goes over wiping her hands on her dress or apron, speaks to Syd on the phone in the kitchen in the near dawn, I'm looking for an exit, wondering how Syd will handle this one, feeling terrible for all of us, wanting to leave and not be seen again . . . she comes off the phone unexpectedly fast, talks to me as if none of this has happened. I leave afterwards, somehow Syd's wife becomes my stepmother and Syd becomes my father, I avoid him in this urban sort of town, citylike . . . I think he's drunk but he really isn't, I feel bad to talk to him, just want to go away from them all . . . I am too different from them, they could never understand my life. At the top of a large large hill, a little black kid is running around . . . I steal some things or find them or am given them, run down the hill fast, round the corner, my dad's sitting there, almost leave again thinking he'll be drunk and nasty, he isn't, he looks at me with a calm sadness, we exchange soundless words . . .

(evening)
. . . in realizing how much I love him, the horrible sense in leaving . . .

All things passing, all things coming to ends, more things beginning, soon themselves to seek or grow towards some kind of end, as if all things are made up of some inner core, some seed as that which lies within the heart and ticks away more and more faintly towards its own discreet and particular end, as if the seed is made of stones like those shaped and worn smooth by the sea, by the shift and roll of sands, by the coarse air and the smooth heels of vagabonds, by the passing of so many feet, so many miles, so many days . . . Ah these sunsets and sunrises, dawns and dusks that pull so much from our eyes, from our foreheads and arms growing soft and furrowed beneath age. And tell me for what reason the animal body passes through these tall grasses, along the ledges and windows of day and night, why these leaning red flowers still opening and closing with the wind and the night, why these silver images flickering from far windows down through the alleyways, why this sense of solitude in rooms filled with people, why the sense of loneliness as arms stretch away from the body of a lover, why these quiet moments of desperation along the coast, the standing platform on the wall of the sea, the shift of sands and winds, the continual rippling of waters, the indigo that claims it all—water wind sea skies and the deepest corridors of the heart—just one reason I can claim for my own, one sound of syllables that will press like dampened cloth against sweating brows, why these battle-fields of dreams, these wounding nights and sleeplessness, these steel car-riages that carry us to and away from the sun, the howling dogs down by the dumps, the fagged ones limping through busy thoroughfares, why these senses of grayness that pierce arrow swift along so many visual regions, why these clocks on everyone's arms, why these calendars along endless cheap room walls, why these philosophies emptying characters of armor and dreams, why these foolish characters along every age, why the thrust of senses, acceleration of the heart in so many cities, why the beginning and end of savage desires, why the light in the eyes that passes in time, why the sense of touch on one's shoulder that eases into familiarity, why never the constant and furious sense of loving for all time in all places and endless, totally end-less, why these nations and borders and coincidences, why these moments passing into hours and unfurling like flowers into hideous days of ending, why these ends, these passings, why.

May 7, 1979

Dreams in the last month have been like slides clacking into an old viewer snap snap snap—scenes characters associations life—rhythms reasons forms all change fast.

In this one I was in a shadow-filled house more than a two-story ram-shackle suburban monolithic structure—wood walls floors doors—old but preserved enough to lend an old-styled grace and beauty. They have come to the house: Your son has arrived. I'm startled; didn't know I had a son. It's actually a whole glad rush of senses and I can't wait to see him. Steve, my brother, is there; he tells me that my son is outside will come in shortly. I see this little kid about eleven years old maybe a lot younger maybe nine years old with slightly dirty blond hair. A kid, I suddenly feel grabbed in the heart happy as hell that he's actually my son. Don't remember having a son and with whom. Kid comes into house running around through rooms in particular kid play, attention's diverted constantly by shape and move-ment of world. I avoid him for as long as possible because suddenly I realize I don't know his name, don't want to hurt him by asking him what his name is, after all, I'm his father!! I ask people, What is his name? No one answers and I get increasingly upset though I don't show it outwardly. I go up to Steve, the kid has come in and is over against a far wall sitting on a ledge over a group of reaching people. I ask Steve again and he bends over to my right ear and whispers the boy's name. I realize suddenly I am somewhat deaf in my right ear and I keep asking him to repeat the name. Finally I say, Tell me in my left ear, I can't hear you in this one. He bends like a doctor and starts examining my bad ear. I'm getting frustrated as hell, I wanna talk to my son but have to know his name. Finally he tells me the kid's name is Hun or Huné. Huné is name of bookshop in St.-Germain. Hun is the Attila I've been reading about in Tares(?) history book. I think Huné is more gentle so I go over toward where my son sits, feel all this love for him and it's awkward. He looks up from playing with his fingers and a shyness comes over him: this is his dad he's heard about. We talk a bit and he jumps down from ledge and both of us stroll outside making loose talk, he has some drawings he was working on . . .

I'm in what seems like a Goodwill store looking over racks of coats trying to find a nice jacket—leather or denim—to trade for this big lumpy coat with hood that Pat & J.P. bought for me for Xmas. I hate the thing, want something lighter and sans hood so I can move without feeling like second grader all puffed up in clumsy coat pushed out the door into the world while everyone else has coats they feel comfortable in. I suddenly realize it's a police station, all these men on benches being booked and fingerprinted for unknown "crimes." I go over to a wall rack, pick a coat, a man comes over and hands me a stupid coat with a hood. I say, Naw man I don't want another coat like that, I hate that kinda shit. Wake up.

May 31, 1979

Felt the strangest I've ever felt—leaving Paris tomorrow for New York— did a half-ditch attempt at cleaning up the apartment, packing, sorting out memories of all of this. Brian went out in the afternoon to look for a gift for

Donna. I sat here in the gray light, sudden downpours, clearing, typing out on a piece of paper a good-bye letter to Jean-Pierre. In the middle of it, kids in the school yard screaming, I broke down swiftly—last week of stunned sense in leaving, all of it came out, wailed over them fuckin' type keys, flashed on Normandy and night J.P. went back to Paris, me typing the weekend out on paper to avoid emotional scenes in solitude, it happened anyway. Trying to keep the fucking letter simple, telling him over and over what I feel for him as a human being, dog barking at me 'cause I'm crying, later Brian came home with a PARIS scarf for Donna: It's got a metro map on it so she won't get lost when she comes. I took off, went to the jardin, walked around for ten minutes or so, felt so displaced, wondering why these fucking experiences come, how important is the growth when it's gotta come to an end, seeing so suddenly my faults laid bare, how I coulda done it all differently.

By the time I get it together will things remain the same—wanting to come back to him, how long will it take, basing hopes on future things, doing something as a writer that makes it possible? Am I fooling myself? I ain't capable of pulling my energy together and being a banker or slick-suit businessman, doing anything flashy for big bucks, just dunno how, don't wanna know how and yet there's a big fucking landmass and waterways to get through to even see him again for a *long* period of time. On metro up to Pigalle saw a guy with his shirt unbuttoned to the waist with a huge prison tattoo of a crucified Christ, done with pins and ink, amazing head with blood pouring out and malformed chest and arms. Pigalle newsstand—major drug scenes/exchanges going on. Toothless hoodlum rushing back and forth. Transvestites waving from third-floor windows at me to come up. I feel rearranged.

Went with J.P. late in the night to the room on Bourdonnais to drop off some things of his there. I feel kinda weightless like in any such transition period only worse than ever, weightless and sad and removed as if everything was rushing by me. I thought of past scenes, everything flashing as we moved through the streets in the auto, flashes of the sense in which I've been involved with him. We got to the room. I had the note that I'd typed out to him alone, with the snake rock I'd done in Normandy, the one I had done for myself. Only thing I could think of to give him as I know he liked it and it represented something important to me/of me that I could hand to him. We unpacked the boxes of food and pots and pans, clothes, kitchen utensils, coffee grinder, etc. I slipped the wrapped stone and letter onto the table. He found it there after a while and looked at me: Is this for me? Yeah, I said and laid out on the bed, the mattress under the window holding a dark sky with no stars. I felt tense and beautiful and vulnerable and sad. I thought of plane crashes and endings, the bloodlessness of my once loving arms, a deep sleep something warm and enveloping to make me forget . . . I watched his back, his hidden side illuminated in the small wall lamp's light, he read for a long time, I wondered if he didn't understand what I had written, if the language was too difficult, he turned finally after slowly folding up the letter, noiselessly and deep in thought, he turned and said, It's beautiful and it makes me feel strange. We embraced and held each other as strongly as possible. He lifted up his head and looked me in the eyes and said, I never told you how much I love you because I was afraid to make it too heavy. I thought you might one day leave and I didn't want it to be difficult. I held him and felt such a harsh love for him, a thick fist rising in my heart, he said, You know I'm sad you go back to America, but I'm happy. I'm happy I had the chance to love you for this time. You are . . . We wept on each other's shoulders and made a slow love together for the last time, just being with him for those last hours made me feel better, knowing that I would have an hour or so in the morning with him kept me from any kind of craziness.

June 1, 1979

Morning we woke together and I made coffee while he shaved. We sat and talked quietly while Brian slept. Talk was difficult as we knew for the first time so clearly where we stood in regards to one another. 9:00 rolled around. He got up to leave and we embraced and I walked him to the elevator and it surged, fucking hot tears coming up from my passioned insides, constricting throat, touched each other's hands as the elevator door was closing. His face was white. I wept in the bathroom in a towel to cut the noise. Pat and Jean

Pillu arrived from Germany. More crying. Realizing how much I love Jean-Pierre, how much I love Pat and how beautiful she's been towards me. How well she understands my senses at this point especially concerning Jean-Pierre.

Arrived at Kennedy Airport around 11:30 P.M., got through customs without having to open my bags. A relief. Walking through the building while Brian watched the bags. I passed a bunch of kids, the unsettling subtle violence of New York/America and yet that realization not easing the sense of almost horror at being once again part of the place. Took a sixteen-dollar cab to Brooklyn Heights to Court Street. Standing on the street while cabbie waits and Brian rushes up to one A.M. household to get money for tip, two Brooklyn rowdies walked by shouting jive shit—bebop clatter familiar sounds, big ego in the face of awesome shit of being New Yorkers with bleak chances at life in this society. Almost passed out, felt hot and dizzy and weary and sick of all these huge looming flashbacks into states of past mind, things in the past, attitudes here in America, working for livelihood, the flash lighting of Pizza stand clattering character, dark night over grainy red buildings' rooftops, the glimmer of the chrome in windows, the Yemen Club sign, the cabbie asking me was I a Yemen: You a refugee? Where's Yemen? What's a Yemen?

Cried awhile when I lay down on the mattress Brian laid out on the floor, lying there, dim lights from tree-filled building, grainy light like a film made of New York traffic Expressway sounds, the smell of the four cats in this apartment (Chuckie's place), the horrible sense of weariness from over a day's nonsleep the flight the dislocation from the familiar, all that I've come to accept as home and lover and living—realized I needed some sleep, so slept.

here is this person who sits
in a chair nearing the specific age of
twenty five on a baking august day in nineteen seventy nine in new york city and he
wonders at the loss of control in any sense
of... a man from paris france three feet
from his right thigh dials a number on a black
telephone and this person thinks of periods of
time and movement where he thought love
was two bloodstreams running immeasurably from
the quiet spaces of an auto between roads on
a highway - the sense of loving is no longer
a real thread held in time or in a place
where tan cows low behind tin sheds in
the foggy night. the sea was once cerulean
and beautiful while mythological animals were
carved on the shore among still wet sands
behind by another evenings tides. Moons no
rise above stray dog hills and rivers of so
no longer drift in an aimless and less co
space, a series of games played in urban
each less real than the other, dreaming ceas
be journeys but wakes up hot and covere
with sweat, the body lies rigid and ther
there are sirens out in the massive
streets, car horns and people waiting to
be saved in innumerable startings across
landscape.

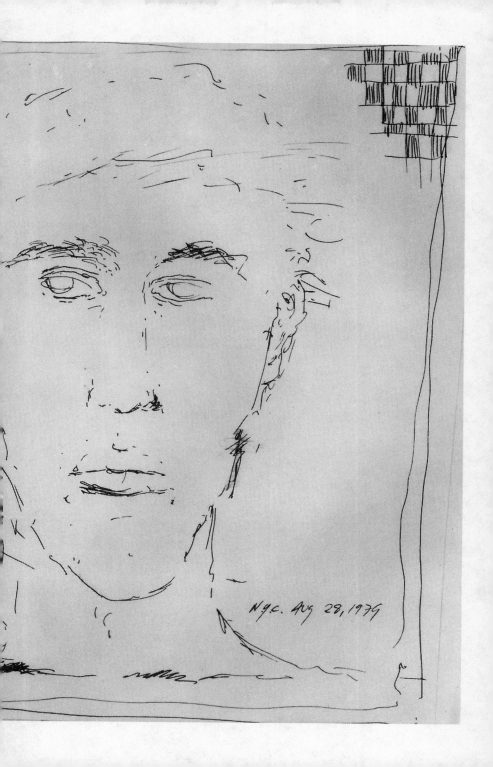

N.Y.C. Aug 28, 1979

Back in New York, David continued to pursue getting his writing published. Much of the journal writing at this time chronicles his sexual experiences on the Westside piers. He started making work using photography and drawing.

June 5–August 28, 1979

June 6, 1979

Brian and I went over to the West Village. So many things to write about, the immediate visual effect of the West Village after nine months in Paris/Normandy. First off (in Dennis's words) it was like an outdoor whorehouse. It's fine to be in a whorehouse when you want to go with a whore but ya don't wanna live in a whorehouse. Now days later, after those first effects I feel a bit more comfortable. Don't think I'll ever forget that initial sense of shock.

Later we walked on down to the Bank Street Pier after stopping in a groceria near 8th Street and getting a couple of containers of carryout coffee. Walked along the West Side Highway structure, roaring autos and grainy darkness, filthy streets with the tugboat strike, a few transvestites out hooking in the shadows of the girder stanchions, a black well-dressed dude pulling down the window of his lit Cadillac as some trans-hooker leans over with a side smile to talk business. Walked out onto the darkened pier, lights on the Jersey shore, the sound of traffic receding at our backs into a shushed roar like faraway ocean or the sense of sound when you're in a bus on a highway and the lid's closing: sound moves around and is heard at a distance. Sat on the end of the pier, the flashes of memories actions scenes past, remembered giving Brian a back rub here one night or was it vice versa? Some guy giving another a blow job on the side strip of the pier. Gave Brian a massage, drank from our coffee containers, talked loosely but mainly laid back in the calm of the night, the moving Hudson River at our backs and sides. Some kinda security as in removal, movements of lights coiling and fracturing on the dark surface of the water, looking back through the darkness towards the skyline, Empire State Building, shafts of illuminated sides of darkened windows, spheres of luminous streetlamps, barely illuminated water tanks, the moon half full and blazing out there in its loneliness: some kind of barometer of the senses depending on time and distance you feel. Normandy moon has a clear foreign sense. New York City moon not so remote and wondrous.

Later heading back we walked along the highway, the motorheads from the cycle bars spilling out in beery crowd onto the streets. Musclemen packed into tight T-shirts and this one albino kid about nineteen or twenty flirting with some of them as he walked in front of us. A group of ten transvestites sitting on car hoods or standing by the sides of gleaming autos, fixing their faces, powdering noses, rubbing on lipsticks and showing each other their clothes, bending down into car mirrors to work with cosmetics. Couple of more reserved joes hanging out with them staring around and looking a bit faded.

Earlier when we went into Tiffany's, a new New York dive restaurant, who was sitting at the counter but the stripper from Paris I talked to in the Tuileries. Blew me away, in fact wish it hadn't happened. Strong wounded senses came up. Thought of Paris and all that I left behind. Disorienting, to say the least. He and I exchanged hellos, he thanked me for writing the letter for him to the strip joint in order to work there again. They took him back. I couldn't say very much to him; it was like all this energy of Paris and the life there: the relationship with Jean-Pierre and all my conflicting desires to return to New York or remain there, my desire now to go back and forget about America (the difficulty in that, especially with my intense love for western landscapes and for friends like Brian). I sat down after mumbling a loose good-bye and dug into some horrible cherry pie and coffee with Brian who was laughing sympathetically, saying, That happens to me all the time.

July 6, 1979

Esther's cousin fell through again; I'd woken up late in the afternoon and talked with Brian after he called Jo-Jo about it. John H. came over in the evening just in time for some hot spaghetti and cheesecake that Brian fixed up and afterwards Brian stayed to do the Edwin story and John and I took the train into Manhattan, I was decked out in my black pants and tuxedo jacket and guerrilla T-shirt and engineer black boots, same thing I had worn at Hurrah's but sans the grease in the hair. We got off in the Village and walked around the streets a bit, I made a couple phone calls to Dirk but he wasn't home, we walked down Christopher Street in the night, crowds of bar characters, homeless cowboys and street sleepers, the roughneck crowds and the junkies on the stoop next to Boots & Saddles and the dollah joints ooo-eee good shit here now dollar joints, mesc, etc., etc. Passed the Silver Dollar with the semitransvestites primping in the side mirrors, day-old leather guys lounging in plastic seats and across tables, pointed the joint out to John as the place that was my usual stomping grounds during the Willy Street period, bands of transvestite gangsters and sleepless days and my head dropped down on greasy slick counter at odd moments in the night till the surreal roar of garbage truck dawn creeping up and that was when the joint changed from sleaze scenes into somethin' like pre-Montana truck stop dives on the faraway road, truck drivers roar up pumpin' brakes and shakin' heads wired with beauties and sliding sideways into the Silver Dollar to seat themselves before plates of steamin' eggs and ham and steaks and cast questioning looks around cluttered tables, at the stragglers from last night's motion . . . every so often this fat queen dancer would tip the bucket and go outta her gourd and wave a small pistol around and wanna shoot up her cheatin' "husband" endin' up in some rat dusty dive behind the door in the eight-by-twelve-foot room weepin' in the soiled mattress and waitin' for him to show his face in the door so she could shoot it up . . . that was a blow to our robbery plans, no one else we knew with enough class to own a gun . . .

Turned the corner at Badlands bar and walked uptown, racing night traffic and glitter of lamps and glass broken on the street and the tittering of transvestites in front of Peter Rabbit bar and the ocean roll of traffic and hiss of wheels the shoooosh of bypassing autos and the glimmer of the river not too far away—we crossed and took various pisses and sat on the water-front board walk and watched the characters easing in and outta the shad-ows of the pier warehouses, along the brick walls like rats and emerging into the phosphorescent shine of bathing streetlamps along the lapping posted walls through various darkness and passing no one—once inside it was difficult to see, a few dim shapes of white T-shirts or the pale gleam of white skin in the darkness, and standin' still for a while our eyes adjusted and we walked toward the back of the pier warehouse where there was one middle doorway shining with a contained section of river and lights, we passed back, John said it was hard to see the ground, we moved directly in the center of the doorway line, seeing two bright spherical yellow lights like car headlights anchored on Jersey cliffs sending vertical lines of light, gold breathin' light across the surface of the dark rolling river, like two railroad track lines laid out into some hobo's heaven, what was that song: Bring me to that place where beef stews grow on bushes, where whiskey trickles from mountain rocks, lemme get that last train, last train (some song from depression hobo repertoire), jokin' to John that it's a giant Chevy parked against the Jersey coastline, images come from the river, the solitude and great sense of foreign remote excitement, all road images coming back from distant places and watchin' these ferryboat barge ships drift by with loud echoing rollin' music coming from their stompin' interiors, part party people on a late-night drift, we turned and walked back in the deep darkness of the pier warehouse and stood against a side wall talking quietly and watching the movements of anonymous characters driftin' back and forth and up and down staircases against the back wall, occasional voices from upstairs and then we strolled back out and onto the bank street pier and towards the end of the pier, avoiding the large gaping holes that open onto the river, my foot almost disappeared down a large pipe aperture, over to the side materializing in the darkness were two men, one giving the other a desperate blow job, Jesus, I said, and John went, Whew . . . and further on were two men one bent over getting rammed by another guy, the fucking was brutal and fast and almost violent but both were into it and then at one point the guy getting rammed was rammed so hard he flew over and his palms landed on the surface of the pier boards and he continued in that position and I just recalled that before in the warehouse we were upstairs walkin' around through hallways and rooms and there was this guy who slid outta the dark and had his shirt removed and positioned himself on the wall and then slid after us as we moved along, he rushin' from door to door and leaning back to caress his chest and crotch and I asked John would he mind waitin' a little bit to the side in the main large room, he did and I went in after the guy, he turned from the wall and ran his tongue over his lips, could feel the dryness of them just by lookin', he whipped out this bottle of amyl and held it under my nose and groped me and I rubbed his chest, his nipples, and he moaned in that hollow darkness, held the amyl under my nose and I placed my hand behind his neck to draw him down to his knees but he turned and slipped away into the darkness and disappeared—I went back to John and we split into a series of rooms windows bordering the river and four perfect diamonds of exterior lamplights laid out on the floor, if ya stand in the middle of the side doorway and walk forward the doorframe empty of door evolves into another room with diamonds of gold light with shadows crossing window frames into another doorway you're still moving forward it's like a film, another set of diamonds on another floor, and the tips of each set of light diamonds appearing less and less in each room, easin' into full view as ya pass forward, eyes on one spot in the unseeing distance, moving like you're on rails—everything relegated to the senses, use of sense like a vehicle, moving forward at regulated pace, something otherwise so unexplainable yet the wounding nature of these visual scenes . . . we watched on the bankstreet pier the fucking until the guys separated and went their various ways, we sat on the far edge next to lapping water and posts and talked about the sense ya get in these scenes that although it's public sex ya still have the sense that ya should respect their privacy and not go over and watch, though watching from a discreet distance can only be expected as it is an intense visual to be confronted with and then another boat went by with characters milling and shoutin' in the din of music, you could barely make out their voices—and the timeless photographical nature of the scenes way back at the beginning of the pier, the trucks lined up silver and motionless, the numerous autos from Jersey and other parts all filled with motionless drivers waiting for someone of their private dreams to walk along softly and open the side door with a click and slide heavy and denimed into the front seat and the pale flash of belly and the motion of the tongue and the slide of hands and the sleeplessness of it all, the bright lights and lampposts burning continuously beneath the Westside Highway structures, the trucks barreling downtown and the two smokestacks to the side in a factory building, squealing autos and the light pale rise of smoke . . . John said as he turned to me that in the pier he experienced some intense excitement, sexual excitement as I did and that in all his fantasies in regards to making love with a guy, maybe not all his fantasies, but in the culmination of them he wanted to make love to me and I felt speechless and yeah felt the pitch of excitement and the newness of it, the whole surrounding sense of making it with a friend I've known for years and traveled with thousands and thousands of miles across the continent and rode freights with in airy Montana mornings, hitchhiking through rolling corn and wheatfields of that Minnesota evening, just at dusk and the bobbing of road lines from stoned vehicles of our past and then it's funny how memory gets the better of us at times and rearranges all events and distorts senses in a way as to clear out things and make room for the important sensory scenes, no, John didn't say all that just yet, we were still getting out of the pier we walked back along the highway towards Christopher Street, against a doorway were five transvestites all yakkin' away done up in their personal glories with makeup and low-cut blouses and silicone shots or hormone tits and John was awed that they were really transvestites and we walked up the stretch of Christopher Street, stopped in the Silver Dollar and ordered coffee and Cokes and toasted English muffins and I called Dirk five times all the time busy on the phone and after that we walked up over to Tenth Street and rang his buzzer and he let us in. A historical moment I proclaimed to them both after getting stoned on some strong weed of John's and Dirk said, What, and I said, Hell, to finally get you two in one room, John as soon as he got there made a dive towards the record collection and started speedily pulling out albums and puttin' them on the side and Dirk stood back and watched everything— Dirk was in a low-key energy but after a half hour was zoomin' right in there, we all got wired on the smoke and Dirk ran through his slides, lotta new ones in there among the ones I saw recently most being time-exposure stuff with televisions waved around in the dark and then flash added to the final fixture of a scene, shots of Suicide and Jackie Curtis and others, the weed was potent and Dirk played sections of records, some L.A. bands and some eastern bands and he and John yakked high-speed about various musics and musicians and their tribe from the no-wave circuits and Dirk on James Chance: He gets us impatient with our impatience for freedom, gets us to feel and gets seized by our impatience for freedom by doing exactly what he wants to do, Sorta Nietzschean, said John . . . listening to PIL's reggae sounds, and the discussion ensued of the quality of the stuff, the ideas of Johnny Lydon creative abilities and flashback to my and John's conversation the other day on the breakup of new no-wave bands and the fact that they appear so fast that there's no disappointment when a breakup occurs 'cause the members of the band that were really putting together stuff will go on and re-form bands and nothing gets stale, the whole idea of no wave being one in which staleness should never will never occur, and if it does occur then it's a defeat . . .

July 6, 1979 (cont.)

Later John went into the bathroom and Dirk set me up on the wall to photograph my T-shirt and tux jacket and stuff with flashlights in semidarkness and color slides, the swirling of camera lens around the flashlight and then delayed flash and captured image of body and shirt and hand and light and then in the bathroom against the black walls and white tiles of the wall next to the sink, I showed Dirk my childhood trick of placing my chin over my shoulder bone and leaning back the displaced sense of body rearrangement and he got weirded out: Ugly, and snapped some shots, got an idea from his cheap toilet paper of wetting and applying it like papier-mâché and covered a side of my face, mouth, and one half of my glasses and went out while the two of them were in conversation and sat on bed till John turned and saw it and giggled and Dirk said, Oh god, and then more photos, one of John holding a white square board like some Devo-esque teacher from the recent future, then a shot of me against the board as John holds it, kinda like exhibit A or B or Z . . . we left afterwards and ate in Tiffany's coffee shop with this bullheaded waiter who had perfected the art of being bored and exasperated, rolling of eyes and long sighs and all as he took our order and served us the stuff, three no-wave women behind us in the next booth with black short razored hair and gold-black circles around their eyes and

cheap plastic black-and-white bulby earrings and sleazo clothes, neat lookin'
and they left after flashin' us some lingering stares, over to the other side in
a booth were two women on quaaludes nodding out over eggs and toast,
chewing with eyes closed for minutes at a time, and the rattle of cars on the
street, the crowds drifting by, one girl who was stunned tripped and dropped
her radio which shattered into various pieces and got up smiling and walked
on . . . we headed for the river afterwards and this was where along the bank
street pier that John said what he felt and I felt nervous as hell, the whole
rearrangement of the way I have always related to him, explained some of
it to him, he was nervous too, of course, as I could imagine, but my senses
got intense and it felt like the first time I'd ever been moving towards a
sexual scene, pit in my stomach tightening up and the racing of senses—we
walked back along the docks and reentered the pier warehouse and moved
to the back and stood in the darkness, all along the walls the sides of the pier
opened out like loading and unloading dock doorways and sections of the
cold night river shimmering and breezing along and every so often the slow
swing of illuminating car lamps from the distance entering the warehouse
and playing over the interior walls, lighting up sections of fallen boards and
glass fractured and scattered along the ways, the slow calm movement of
water, the shudder of it beneath the wind, the crosscurrents whirling into
knots and the sight of city streets and highways and lampposts glittering in
the far-off night and landscape and John said, Ya know, David, I really wanna
kiss ya, and I said, Whew, and stood there dumbly for a second and then
abandoned the nervousness best as I could and we kissed and then embraced
and felt my hands running smooth over his jacket then sliding beneath the
jacket under his shirt over his shoulders while his hands touched various
parts of my back and ran along and we stopped for a breath, the disordering
of past senses, the idea of images blown away as in an earlier conversation
along the river wall on the side of this warehouse, in a manmade cove of
warehouses and he talked about last night at Hurrah's dancing with me and
with Brian and the sense of blowing the ideas contained in being friends,
the intense symbolism of removing ties of fear, the real sense of it as emergence into new areas and explorations and jesus the exciting prospects and
possibilities contained in that kinda action . . . I had a copy of William

Burroughs's *The Algebra of Need* balanced on the ledge of the closed unloading dock door next to where we stood as we started getting it on we
got involved, the situation becoming more and more intense and hot, the
idea that if I was ever gonna make it with a guy that I loved and knew previously as a traveling buddy that this place in the predawn hours had to be
the one right place in this fuckin' city to do it, the sense of foreign displace-
ment in accordance with my body and mind, the environment following
with the change of head, and I lifted up his shirt and kissed him on the chest
and ran my tongue down his sides and around his neck and felt with my
palms and fingers all around his legs and back and face and it got more intense till we knocked off the book from the ledge and it slammed with a
loud bang on the floor, soon after there were voices, sounded like tough
rip-off characters, a small gang of voices, the projection of fear in the form
of cut throats, we stood there in the darkness rearranging our shirts and jackets
and pants, zipping up and buckling up and listening for the direction of their
voices, high-pitched pseudofeminine shrieks asking indecipherable questions, the mal intent contained within the sound finally we eased outside
into the river walkway, walked frantically back and forth trying to figure
how to get away or what to do, the voices looming suddenly real close and
we sat down against the door where moments before we'd been on the other
side: Imagine a force field, a field of protective energy, our heads ran away,
the slow dawn was beginning to be apparent on the outer traces of horizon,
I was thinking mass energy, white fields of light, protective energy, the voices
got closer, felt claustrophobic on the edge of the great river on the edge of
the great city, massive distances come and gone, the great endless sky and
felt claustrophobic like, no place to run, they finally came tittering out a
number of yards away, a bunch of queens looking for people fuckin' around,
bored of waiting endless hours in the upper-floor corridors for the necessary animal embrace, they came down looking for it, looking to disrupt it if
possible and guess they didn't see us—they rattled around the walls for a
while, giggling and shrieking and John and I sighed and laughed quietly
and realized the projection of fears in our heads, and yet the possibilities it
could've been, talked about throwing them in the river were we to start
fighting, jumping in ourselves if need be, finally walked around inside looking

for a quiet place to get it on, went out the back of the wall door and stretched out on the asphalt of the dock and talked and smoked a cigarette and I ran my hand over him and stretched out and then the dawn was on its way up with lightening colors of sky, a rusty tinge of red-orange coming up behind the factory across the way, the one past the next pier, the two simultaneous stacks almost merged with one another in the perspective of sight and growing a brown brick color, emerging from the darkness into the coming dawn, shadows slowly easing away, the water with small almost indiscernible flickering lines, like schools of fish just beneath the surface racing along and surging but not yet moving further but where they were, turmoils of water, and easing his pants down we looked over our shoulders and there was some young guy standing there surveying the scene like we weren't part of it, how long he was watching I don't know but with a weary shake of heads we got up and readjusted our clothes and slipped back into the warehouse, walked around a bit, watched the intense visuals of dawn, the elevated structure of the Westside Highway and the burning lampposts, the incineration of the dawn, the backdrop domelike sky over the city lightening and the water turning to an azure blue, to turquoises and silvers, the merging of blood rust reds into the surfaces as if dawn were a flaming vehicle come rolling down across the plains and highways to step slowly into the river of time, the Indian giver of moments, the pulling in and the pushing forward, the continuance of senses, the changes that have rolled up and in and pulled me along since my return from the quiet city of Paris, the lonesome city and the darkness that shuts off my sense of abandonment in that faraway place—we walked into the back part of the warehouse, outside where the cove was, the U-shaped arena of warehouse walls and windows, along the ledge where there was miraculously some kinda cheap rug, dollar a yard kinda rug stretched over the ledge and dry and we lay down and watched the dawn rising in the windows and whole landscapes emerging from the disappearing night, the burning of lampposts in the now gathering dawn and somewhere out there were two huge metal barges filled with stuff I couldn't make out, bobbing and drifting in the river as huge waves pulled in from passing tugs and barges and small ships and the moon long gone and the open doorways of the warehouse across the way revealing orange vehicles, trucks and forklifts and crates and still burning lights and John asked me to stand up after I caressed him and ran my mouth and tongue over his chest and down into his belly and further down as I pulled his pants back and I stood up and the dawn light was intense, the revelation of the night before, the landscapes we'd drifted through, the zombie presence of men drifting back and forth in the dispelling of Rechy's myth that dawn was the quietest hour when all cruising ended and streets were empty, he embraced me kneeling down and I felt hot streaks of excitement rising up and over-powering my limbs, felt weak and dizzy both of us at times did, felt awed by the placement of ourselves in this light, the sense of his mouth warm and smooth, hands sliding over bare legs and somewhere in those moments I came and felt totally drained of all energy and tension and wanted to drop to my knees and lie there thinking for hours on end, instead we arranged our clothes and sat down and lit a cigarette and mused out loud about the last fifteen hours or so and the sense of life and loving and explosion of images and experiencing of senses . . . the world trade center, the very top of it emerging into a dim sunlight of rising dawn, it was framed by crossbars of metal on top of the far warehouse roof and it was like some kinda vision in all of this, in this morning and night and actions and touching and senses allowed to surface in long continual slides of motion . . . we sat there talk-ing about both of us and Brian and the things we'll someday do in the form of street actions and creative energies and maybe ultimately in the form of band work, the sexual senses in growing up, the pleasurable scenes in the night and dawn, the senses of ourselves with women, the continuation of the senses in that, the pleasure of various acts and movements and some-where along the way we rose up and entered the warehouse and went back upstairs and walked the hallways and the rooms and the group of queens who had disrupted us before sat around on the floor and left as we entered and somewhere in there someone said, David, and I turned and it was some guy I once knew and had written something for and never bothered to see again after my return for unknown reasons, and we left finally and walked over to Sheridan Square to a coffee shop and had breakfast and talked of dis-eases and of other things and then hit the subway and went our separate ways and crashed in our own ways in our own homes in our own beds and slept.

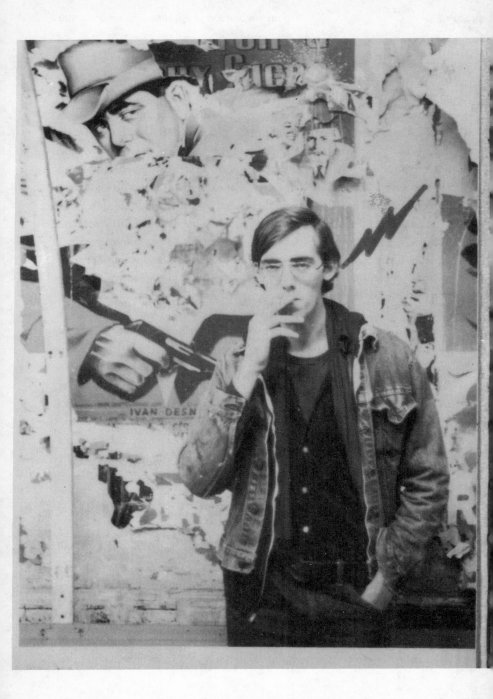

October 8, 1979

Visited the river again this evening, red traces of dusk far behind the sea green walls of Jersey shipping warehouses, red aura glow inside the pier warehouse walking from room to room, dusk through busted walls getting cruised by lanky queens, searching for the man from Texas, looked through the blue night halls, the warm rooms with pale filmic images of men in boots fucking other men in corners, the ghosts of leather jackets and boys with pasty faces behind concrete walls slow movements extending from shoulder to elbow to wrist, drifting images of desire range rogue desire in the irises immersed in shadow like the folds of river water over the face, seas in fading light, the dead man falling fathoms, the live man falling fathoms, the long lingering sight, the stare into folds of depth of unbreathing moisture, the erotic sense of withdrawal behind misty walls of concrete, the image of sense seen in their eyes not invisible to me, the scene obscured by walls and shadow, the man from Texas wasn't there. I drifted, turned on heel in doorways, lit matches to give sparks to cigarettes, pushed away hands, walked the stone cliff walls of the warehouse exterior and made my way into a bar on the waterfront down the highway. The first few minutes being confronted with exciting images and realizing them to be false, to be costume and pose, to be nonexistent in such environments. Realizing with the Texan man, the sense he evoked in the meeting, the senses I've been left with that are a bit unsettling, unsettling in their intoxicating beauty, in their rarity, the sense that I'd gladly give this stranger my soul my life my time in movement in living for the rest of my life, would live with him immediately, the giving away of preoccupation or routine to be finely held in the mind and rough hands of a stranger, this produced in the meeting a series of movements along

a darkening hall, the heavy sound of footsteps, the casual swagger of a character turning on the silent balls of his feet, the motion toward me erasing
the definition of "stranger" making us less than strangers, the cocking of his
head to the side, healthiness of the light in his eyes, the broad face, nose.
How it is I'd give my life for/to him, not a sense of ego or egolessness, my
life being very important to me in personal freedoms, but like riding in a
truck through the images of Texas, the badlands, the rolling vistas the buttes
cactus and fine sands of timelessness, the ever-present rouge line on metal,
the continuous dusk at our feet, the guns over the visors, the bullets in the
dashboard, the riding riding motion of the senses, realizing the futility of
ever really creating this act, this act of merging physically and psychically
with this man from Texas, the impossibility of it, for in the repetition of
these scenes it would no longer be present, this intoxication, this sense of
unlimited possibilities in the stopping of time and aging this controlled recklessness in pursuit of time distance light and landscape. But still again the
possibility of doing this with this man, doing it or having the sense of being
able to do it only because of the unlikeliness of it ever occurring, like there
is a chance that someday in these New York streets I might bump into him
again and get it on again, get it on in the same ruggedly sensitive way, the
beauty of visuals and all they evoke, what those minutes in the dim dusk
hallway light gave me, what sense of my past and my desires they opened
up. It's the sense of possibility in living life the way I've wanted to live it—
never really having lived the life I've wanted, never having that control of
destinies or scenes or motions or moments, no one ever having that (thus
the excitement in it). Really it's this lawlessness and anonymity simultaneously that I desire, living among thugs, but men who live under no
degree of law or demand, just continual motion and robbery and light
roguishness and motion, reading Genet out loud to the falling sun overlooking the vast lines of the desert receding into dusk and darkness, drugs
and aimlessness, the senseless striving to be something, the huge realization
of the senselessness of that conscious attempt in the midst of the way this
living is really constructed, the word *constructed* not even being sensible,
unreal, the endless forms of chance and possibility as an alternative to construction, the free floating in time/space/image, the futility and impossibil-

ity in even subscribing to the definition of it for even in the definition in the construction of words is the inherent failure to obtain the living sense of the desire. So although I've lived forms of movement that approach or start to come close to the scenes I desire, the life I desire, still when all is said and done, just as in the construction of these words I have still not touched the edge of it. Thus in the visual scenes, the erotic senses evoked by the meeting of this man in the darkening halls of the pier warehouse, in those odd moments where the walls were on fire with the heat of his body, with the heat of his associations headwise and physically, in all of this witnessed by the hermaphrodite along the wall clattering noiselessly into the future on Magic Marker high heels, was I given a reprieve in the impossibility of actually living my life as it should be, as my sensibilities demand, thus the momentary departure into time and distance, the sense of myself living in controlled recklessness within the pure sound embraced by his body and mind as in the uttering of the word *Texas* rolling off his tongue and lips in the change of shadows and light, his eyes perceiving me cast on the fiery night of receding deserts and seas, the motion of the gray river in the rain, the sound of tireless traffic in the wet streets. The possibility inherent in impossibility. The sense of slight chance in a future time when elements fall together in random order providing the entranceway through all of life and death but only with the body so inextricably entwined with the pull of desire and motion and distance that the senses run on a thin wire of fire unstrung, unsung and believable (livable).

October 28, 1979
A.M.

Went to see *Le Prophète* Friday night with Alan at the Met. First opera I've seen. Throughout the performance kept visually rearranging what was taking place onstage, subvocally replacing lines of song with spoken or sung poetics. Wondered at Robert Wilson's *Einstein on the Beach,* how amazing it must have been. *Le Prophète* was pretty boring, realized the singers of the middle-upper-class characters retaining this form through time as something to be indulged in and appreciated in a removed way, small personal pleasures I guess, but more important, how the modernization of such forms could be quite amazing, enthralling, etc. A few moments here or there where the voice was interesting in its sounds, manipulations, otherwise was quite boring. Had to pinch my own leg to refrain from bursting out laughing during solemn scenes. Later showed Alan my artwork. He seemed a bit put on the spot, not wanting to have to tell me he did not like the drawings because of their content. I felt a bit awkward and sad at our obvious differences in perception. It magnified the very things Dirk and I talked about in terms of the conscious choice of imagery we work in, how it becomes unsettling or mildly threatening to those who enjoy an established order or large-scale security. How could I explain that these images reflect energy I've picked up in society, in movement through these times? It's just a translation of what takes place in the world. I found myself almost apologetic because of the choice in what I'd created. Those distances (the horror! the horror!) in between people like me and Alan or myself and Randy or myself and numerous others. At one point after waking I asked him what images would be beauty to him (in response to his question/statement: You have talent, why don't you use it to draw beautiful things?). His descriptions of images were beautiful, I had to agree, they were images to which I'd also be drawn, imagery I hope to put down on paper in the future. But still in all they don't answer my own or other people's questions of why I'm drawn to images that unsettle or confront the viewer in an intense way. I once tried to define it for myself, actually I've made numerous attempts at defining it but all I come up with are somewhat lame quasi-psychological reasonings such as: in opposition to the large period of time in which I hid the actions of my youth, street routines, homosexuality, etc., etc., after age twenty I began showing people my more murderous images or writings as if to shock them, or to introduce to them the things or representations of things I'd always felt pressured to keep hidden, placing my enormous head-held energies into others' hands rather than acting as the silent guard of them.

Don't know if I'll ever come to understand it. But possibly the way forward is for me to try to extend the range of creative acts to cover both images of beauty (silent disturbing beauty) and of intensity—in drawn images and in written images and in photographic images. In doing this—

creating a range rather than keeping the beauty hidden as I have done within journals, head, etc.—then I can at least have the physical proof of that range, and thus no longer feel the need to explain it or prove it in conversations or apologize for not having shown the range in its entirety that I feel is contained within me. Delighting as well as shocking that angel within my forehead.

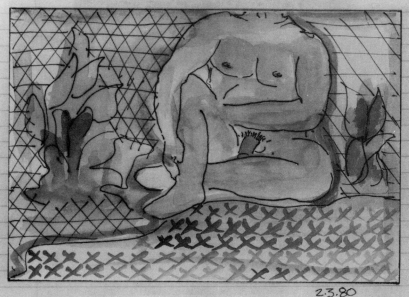

2.3.80

February 4, 1980

Went out walking around the neighborhood along the river where the dark streets are gently illuminated, pools of light slipping down brick and stone and iron walls and easing over the smooth surfaces of cobblestones . . . Met this guy I've seen before. He stopped his car on a side street and rolled down the windows and waved me over, flashing a smile from the darkness of his car's interior. We drove down the hill towards the river, pulled into a vast factory parking lot, an enormous pancake of dirt spread beside the Manhattan Bridge and surrounded mostly by river. The slow lights of barges and the bleak iron giantcy of a crane that in the morning barely after the sun rose would be pummeling away at the hard earth amidst the clang of hammers and cries of workmen— He slid down in front of the seat and worked my belt loose from its loop and placed his smooth hands under my sweatshirt rubbing my chest in circular rough motions. After a while, through the condensation gathering on the cold windows from my heated breath, I saw the familiar blue and white colors of a cop car swing round and bounce over the lip of the parking lot border. They swung towards us as I quickly pulled up my pants and awkwardly fastened the belt. After stopping briefly by our car they continued on to another car parked not far away, the inhabitants of which had been making various photographs of the waterfront and skylines. Then they returned and parked so that their headlights shone in and filled our car with blazing lights. I quickly asked the guy to repeat his name in case we were questioned. He did so and rolled down his window. I could see the cops through the haze of lights crawl from their cars and approach. They shone a high-intensity flashlight into our car and played their rays across our laps. I wondered if my zipper was all the way up, if they would notice the outline of my underwear stretched around my legs. I was ordered out of the car after one cop said, Just looking at the river? I was tempted to say, Whatcha think asshole? but spared the poor guy. I felt simultaneously angry and worried. After a couple seconds I completely relaxed, thought about what was unfolding and realized despite cops and laws, I was doing nothing that I felt was wrong. Immediately I calmed down and the prospect of getting arrested didn't faze me, but I kept my tongue in check for the driver's sake. I got out of the car as the cop demanded, and found it slightly awkward to walk with my underwear impossibly stretched around my calves. The second cop came around to me and both cops simultaneously asked each of us what was the other guy's name. I answered, I think his name is Fred but I'm not sure. Not sure, huffs the stupid cop. Whataya mean, yer not sure? Well, I said, I don't know his name too well. He's just a guy I see every now and then and sit and talk with. The cop looked at me and told me to start walking. I thought I misunderstood him so I asked him to repeat it. He said, Start walking! Go on, get outta here. I went back to the car to retrieve my coat and the two cops got into a bit of an argument, one saying that I could return to the car, the other telling me to walk out of the lot. Finally, one backed down and I was told to start walking, which I did as Fred rolled his car out of the lot. I walked out behind him and he slowed up to ask if I was all right. I answered, Fine. I'm okay. I'll see ya another time up on the hill. With that the cop car speakers crowed out, I TOLD YOU NOT TO PICK HIM UP. NOW KEEP MOVING. I waved good-bye and turned a corner and headed up the hill into the night.

I ran into the old Lithuanian woman who owns the building as I returned home. She was standing far off in the dark field with her two mangy old dogs, two great animals that look like strange Australian desert pigs with hides like the stuff old worn carpets are made of. I walked into the field towards her and said hello. She was rosy-cheeked even in the darkness. She went into a sad monologue about her family in Russia: My brother—I have thirteen brothers and sisters—my one brother just twenty years old refused to go to Siberia so they threw him on a train, very dark and crowded, no windows and no fresh air, nothing much to eat, many other people in the cars, for a long long distance they take him, my father, too. See they come around and say to all these farmers—my father was a very good farmer—these men come around and tell all the farmers to sign a paper that says we have one big farm, but no, we have a whole lot of little farms. Many people say, No, I won't sign the paper. And boom, they are taken away to Siberia, many young children, whole families, fathers, the parents but not the children, or half the family . . . I see my father dragged off to Siberia, where it's very cold and no heat and he dies very quickly there. And my brother, twenty years old, they fire a gun at him. I see his stomach, a big hole opens in his stomach . . .

There's nothing so horrifying as war stories from the mouths of the people who experienced it. Like in Europe, all those people who saw their relatives die . . .

February 8, 1980

Time on the river had become irrelevant—walking down into the darkness of the side streets and avenues, crossing the highway, cars burning in lines going uptown and downtown, waiting beneath the overpass, papers skidding along the loading docks, some character standing beside a solitary car in darkness, over by the river a series of cars easing from parking spots on the asphalt runway, others turning off along the waterfront, circular motions of vehicles, burning headlights acting like beacons that sweep over the surface of the river, the river looks like clouds, the rafts of ice driven together by currents, spread from the shore to the center of the river protected from being swept away by the piers. When the headlights swing away from the surface of the river, everything is settled into a calm easy darkness, ice merges into a slow illuminated color of night, the bare ridges of the ice floes exposed, like arctic childhood memories, waiting for the polar strides and windy howls of desolation.

A large sheet of corrugated iron has been nailed over the walkway that once led to the covered pier. No more scenes there; all of it relegated to the past, summers' movements held in my mind like a series of film clips, the rooms that evolved into rooms, the dusty heat that survived the winds and spread through the structure, sounds of gasping and the slow scrape of shoes across the floors, cinematic motions unfolding before my eyes, scenes of renegade men I had never known, scenes straight from the novel mind, wildboys breathing life, clothes slowly being removed by strangers' hands, the slight breeze drying the sweat of arms and legs and ruffling through the dense hair of sweet crotches. The light aligning itself with motion, curves of legs and arms and upturned necks, the murmur of sensation, dreams uttered from faces with closed eyes. Now just windy noise clashing with silence of night, big tin sheets banging in the wind and dense burnt breezes flowing from shattered windows and twisted roofs, the stars above, the winter still riding over the mouth of the structure, ships still passing ominously in the darkness, lights of the Jersey cliffs burning and winking, a huge cigarlike cloud of steam tilting from the lip of a factory smokestack, the neon red cup of coffee dripping continuously there against the snow-covered rocks of the coast.

A car came circling in from the highway, a pale face turning towards me behind the window, the eyes of the driver shielded in shadow, lips frozen for a moment in motion as the car makes a swift curve somewhere further down and swings back to envelop me in light. I turned and stared at the driver as he swept past, his face turning towards me once again, the invitation in the sudden parking of the vehicle a dozen yards away. I walked around in the cold, moving my hands around within my pockets to warm them, went to the other side of the car and stood there motionless, watching the lower torso of the driver with hands on the wheels. Finally he bent forward, his head came into view, and he peered questioningly at me: a sharp click of the door locks. I went over and opened the door and slid in sideways. He let the light remain on so as to answer some unasked questions and then click, the car was turned towards the night, darkness taking the place of hands and legs and shadows covering our faces. He said he didn't talk English, a slightly familiar accent on his tongue. Qu'est que tu parle? I asked. Ah bon, español, français, etc. We talked in loose French as he swung the car away from the river and drove further down, away from the motion of strangers and the clusters of other cars. He was a slim guy with thick black hair, sweet face belonging to rogues along Pigalle, dense like old photos of Mayakovsky, thick features, nose and lips and cheek-bones formed from some sensual stone. Broad shoulders and a pair of hands that showed muscle and veins in their broadness. He unbuckled my belt in the shadows of the vehicle, thrust his mouth down along the pale area of my exposed stomach, traced lines with his tongue over its curves. Roughly pulling my pants further down around my legs he dipped and licked smooth areas of saliva around the curve of my knees, beneath my knees which drove me wild, in a swift motion releasing his own cock from his trousers and placing my hand upon it. He blew me in a series of rough motions, his tongue darting back up to my abdomen and up across my sides, over my chest, leaving very slight luminous trails across its surface, my hand moistened with my tongue slid back down to his cock and I leaned my head back as he pulled me towards him, murmuring something in French I couldn't understand, feeling him attempting to enter me I came into his curved palm, gasping against the noise of the winds that crashed along the coast.

February 21, 1980

The river was dirty and coming towards me in the wind, a smooth chest trembling with sweat. The movement of him in the bare doorway, green fields opening beneath the moon and the neoned coast. This desire, so small a thing, becomes a river tracing the drift of your bare arms, dark mouth, and memories of strangers. All things falling from the earth and sky: small movements of your body on the docks, moaning down there among the boards and the night, car lights slanting across the distance, airplanes in deep surrender to your rogue embraces. A smile sparking grin, a darkening house, from behind car windows, the moving confidence of transvestites along the highway. The wind plays along the coast sustained by distance and leveled landscapes, drifts around bare legs and through doorways of barrooms. Something silent and recalled, the sense of age in a familiar place, the emptied heart and light of the eyes, the white bones of streetlamps and autos, the press of memory turning over and over and I'm coming. Later sitting over coffee and remembering these cinematic motions as if witnessed from a discreet distance, laying the senses down one by one, writing in the winds of red dawn, turning over slowly into sleep.

February 23, 1980

Standing in the waterfront bar, having stopped in for a beer in midafternoon, smoky sunlight fading in through the large plate-glass windows and a thumping roll of music beating invisibly in the air . . . Over by one window and side wall a group of guys hanging out playing pool, one of them this Chicano boy, muscular and smooth with a thin cotton shirt of olive green, black cowboy hat pushed down over his head, taut neck rising out of the cut of his shirt, strong collarbones pressing out, a graceful curve of muscles in his back and a solid chest, his stomach pressed like a slightly curved washboard against the front of his shirt, muscles in his arms rising and falling effortlessly as he gesticulates with one hand, talking with some guy who's leaning into the sunlight of the window, in his other hand the pool stick balanced against his palm, a cigarette between his fingers. He leaned back and took a drag and blew lazy smoke rings slow one after the other that pierced the rafts of light and dissolved within the shadows. The guy he was talking to looked like some midwestern country boy straight from the fields of gathered wheat and dusty back roads traveled by pickups with beer cans in the backseat and a buzz in the head from summer. He had dark eyes and a rosy complexion, a roughly formed face made of sharp lines and his hair cut short around the sides and back of his neck. Standing there drinking from my bottle I could see myself taking the nape of his neck in my cold white teeth, a shudder of eroticism as he turned and stared out the window for a moment at the traffic. Light curved around his cheeks and the back of his head, the shaved

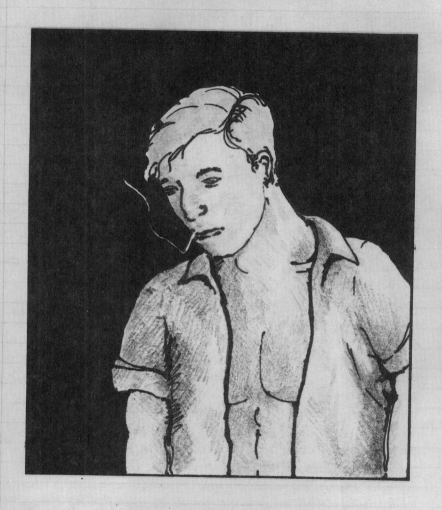

hair having left bristles that I could feel against the palm of my sweating hand, all the way across the room. He looked around after turning away from the window and set his eyes on me for a long moment, studying me for indiscernible reasons, and I felt the bass of the music tapping in on some center where my emotions or passion lies, I tilted my head back and took another swig from the beer, humming gathering from my stomach and rising up around my ears. He turned away and the Chicano guy leaned over the pool table for a shot, his back curved and taut like a bow, arm drawing back to clack the balls softly on the table, a couple dropping into side pockets and for a moment the two of them were lost in a drift of men entering the bar. I moved over a few feet to bring them back in view and some sort of joke had developed between them, the country boy reached into the bottom slot of the table and withdrew a black shiny eight ball and advanced towards the Chicano, who drew back until his buttocks hit the low sill of the window. He giggled and leaned his head back letting a hardness come from his eyes. The country boy's face turned a slighter shade of red, and he reached out with his hands, one hand pulling the top of the Chicano's shirt out, and the other deftly dropping the eight ball into the neckline. The ball rolled down and lodged near his torso and the two of them laughed as he reached in, hand sliding down his chest and stomach I would have readily laid my forehead to, and retrieved the ball. I took a last swig from my beer, overcome with the heat that had been gathering within my belly and now threatened to overcome me with dizziness, barely managed to place the bottle upright on the nearby cigarette machine and push open the doors into the warm avenue winds, push open the doors and release myself from the embrace of the barroom and the silent pockets of darkness and the illuminating lines of light thinking it was Jacques Prevert who said, Why work when you have a pack of cigarettes and sunlight to play with, and listened to the horns of ships along the river, far away over the fields of buildings and traffic, turned a corner and headed crosstown. Pleasure derived as much from the witnessing of lovely images as from any sexual embrace. Remembering how when I was younger and was rejected by the sturdy rogue men ten years older than me whom I met within the dark avenues of the river, how I came close to telling them it didn't matter, I had their images, their faces and bodies and all the associations in my head to go home at leisure and lay down upon the warm sheets of a summer room and lay my hand to myself and have them anyway.

February 26, 1980

Walking down by the waterfront this morning I met the old guy who looks like Jean Genet, grizzled and dirt lines in the creases of his neck skin, vaguely handsome, red print worker's hankie around his throat, shorn hair, white and stubbled. He invited me up to look at his room in the Christopher Street Hotel. Climbed three flights of stairs after passing a clerk's glass booth with a radio playing and no one inside. He turned the key in the lock and the door swung open on a gray dim-lit room about twelve by twelve feet, all over the walls were various gray newspaper photographs torn from dailies and taped up to the peeling paint. Most were photos of President Carter and his wife, and a couple of Carter's mother. Other photos were of American flags, and he also put stick-on flags over each picture, some on a wall calendar, a flag on each month, and a couple lost somewhere in a paint-splashed collage left behind by another tenant. On an old stained mattress which lay on the floor he had his biggest flag, one that covered most of the mattress like a blanket. He showed me a greeting card with some seminude woman like a Vargas *Playboy* painting, over which he'd written a letter to Carter's mother: How do I know if she didn't look like this when she was younger? See, I figured she prolly did . . . that's what I tell her in this letter . . . He gave me a Xeroxed stapled piece, one of his street-Steinian discourses on being an American and loving the country for what it could be. He started rambling about language and writing, how one should write what they speak rather than play with imagination: You stand up and write, ya know . . . standin' up is good for writing because you don't use your imagination, you let come from yourself what would come if you were speakin' to someone . . . when you sit down to write, it's no good 'cause the whole weight of your body centers down in that position, the weight carried by the head, through the head, so you end up writing with imagination instead of natural speech. He kept asking me to sit down, cackling afterwards and saying,

Whatsa matter you afraid I might try and rape ya . . . heh heh. Later he tried explaining some stuff he realized when he smoked weed: When I smoke I get real intense things going on in my head and it wants to bust out so I start writing, that's how it comes out . . . People should sing all the time . . . ya know . . . if you say five words very very slowly then you end up singing . . . if everyone were to speak very slowly then everyone would be singing . . . then things would be nice. How can you be fucked up when you're singing?

February 28, 1980

He had a tough face, square-jawed and barely shaven, tight-cropped hair, wiry and black, intensely handsome like some face seen in old boxer photos of Rocky Marciano, a cross between him and Mayakovsky, a nose that might've once been broken in some dark avenue barroom in the water-front district of a distant city, a slight hump to it, that curved down towards a rough mouth, beautiful lips. Sitting in a parked car by the river's edge he leaned over and placed the palm of his hand by the water, and then placed the palm of his hand along the curve of my neck and stroked it slowly, his hands and arms brown like the skin of his face, a slight tan slowly receding to a blush. The heat was pumping in the car, the waves turned over and over by the coasting wind that shot across the river beneath the darkening clouds. Some transvestites circled down from the highway going from car to car leaning in the drivers' windows to check for business. A couple of trucks from out of state, probably Kansas or Montana or Wyoming, idled near the abandoned warehouse, the interiors cleared of the beef carcasses and the drivers sitting up high in the cabs, the last cowboys with their wives or girlfriends sitting next to them, beehive bouffants and flannel shirts and Saran-wrapped sandwiches and a bottle for comfort. So this guy eases his hand down towards my legs and slides it back up beneath my shirt, says, Take it off, and I reach down and lift the sweaters and sweatshirts up to-gether and pull them over my head and drop them to the floor where my pants are straddling my ankles. He pulls off his olive green army sweater revealing a T-shirt of ice blue, reaches down and lifts that off afterwards, revealing a gleaming torso, thick chest with a smooth covering of black hair, two brick red nipples buried inside the down. He turns and bends over me, licking me softly with his tongue, tonguing smooth circles around my nipples down my sides, his hand massaging slow between my legs, his other hand wetted briefly against his mouth and working his cock up till it's dark and red and hard. When he lifted away from my chest I saw his eyes, the pupils, the irises the color of lapis lazuli dark chips of circular stone, something like the sky at dusk after a clear hot summer day, when the ships are folding down into the distance and dreams are uttered from the lips of strangers and white jet streaks are etched against the oncoming darkness, connecting whole cities with a single line. I could feel myself falling into them, populating them with dense mythologies and histories, quiet green neighborhoods of tree-lined streets and dusty fields left abandoned and long dirt roads that led into time unknown and secrets loosened by the faint roars of sixteen-wheel rigs barreling over the horizon. Whole dark winds rattling over plains be-hind those eyes. Yeah, and he had said he was from the West.

March 6, 1980

Went down to the river tonight speeding again. Had dropped the Eskatrol in the Silver Dollar sometime in the late afternoon before the sun began fading. It was a mixture or rather overlapping of seasons today, almost but not quite mild weather, a cool breeze circling in from the river and enough of a sun to leave my coat open and flapping. Before I dropped the speed I went for a walk along the river, the light so bright in reflection off its sur-face that I had to continually shield my eyes to avoid being run over by the stray cars cruising for drag queens. They were out in force, done up in choice colors and makeup and pacing the parking lots, dipping up and down be-fore the windshields of parked cars looking for a horny laborer or business-man on his lunch hour. Half the cars with Jersey plates, making me wonder how far they've come, what distances traveled and how they saw New York from that other side, realizing Jersey will never change, the symbol of change at some future point will be recognizable when the tan plates stop showing up along the waterfront.

Some guys in the early afternoon in the warehouse were shouting among themselves and stepping forward in the musty interior. I realized they were scavenging the place for pipes containing copper wiring—a few sawed-off pipes jutting from the torn upstairs wall. Down on the main floor they were arguing, three of them, about which pipe length in the maze attached to the dark shadowed ceiling held the power lines for the place. One guy up in the rafters, scaling pipe lengths like a gymnasium, was hanging by his arms with his muscles cording beneath his short sleeves, the front of his sweatshirt riding up his belly and revealing a rippled stomach. From his soot-blackened pants hip he unclipped a hacksaw and began drawing it over a length of the pipe like a violinist, his strong legs swinging back and forth in time to the sawing, almost imperceptibly.

Upstairs some queens were walking amid the charred refuse, picking their way over blackened beams that hung out of the sky alongside twisted iron girders. They had a large black and chrome radio carried by one of the younger members of the group who twirled the station selector back and forth while at high volume so a strange series of voice and music and static bounced in and out of the rooms.

Later at the Silver Dollar restaurant, I sat at the stool counter and ordered a small cola and let the pill ride the tip of my tongue for a moment and then swallowed it. As usual, just as I drop some stuff I have a sudden regret at what will be the disappearance of regular perceptions, of the flat drift of sensations gathered from walking and seeing and smelling, into a strange tremor like a tickling that never reaches a point of being unbearable, a slow sensation of that feeling coming into the body, from the temples to the abdomen to the calves. And riding along with it in waves, I feel the marvelousness of light and motion and figures on the streets. Yet somehow that feeling of beauty that comes rising in off each surface and movement around me always has a mask of falsity about it, a slight sense of regret I feel at the recurring knowledge that it's a substance flowing through my veins that cancels out the lines of thought brought along with my aging and seriousness.

So there's that feeling of regret, a sudden impulse to bring the pill back up, a surge of weariness, then the settling back and waiting for the sensations to begin, wondering what they'll bring. So I dropped this pill and sat there for a while, smoked a fast cigarette and the door opened in the front of the place and some young guy in his midtwenties with racing sneakers and a boomerang curve of red adorning them comes in slinging a small backpack to the floor beneath the counter and slides onto a stool and orders the same as me. Handsome guy with strong cheekbones recalling France and the *jardins* and faces in the slight rain towards evening in the summer. Old images racing back and forth and I'm gathering heat in the depths of my belly, flashes of a curve of arm, back, and the lines of a strong neck belonging to some character among crowds in train stations and I get up, pay for my drink, and start through the door for the first of many walks to come that day. Restless walks filled with coasting images of sight and sound, cars buckling or bucking over cobblestones down quiet side streets, trucks waiting at corners with swarthy drivers leaning back in cool shadowy seats and windows of buildings opening and closing, figures passing within the rooms, faraway sounds of voices and cries and horns that roll up and funnel in like some secret earphone connecting me to the creakings of the city. There's a discreet pleasure I have in the walking of familiar streets, streets familiar more because of the faraway past than for the recent past, streets that I walked down odd times while living amongst them, seen through the same eyes but each time the eyes belonging to an older boy, spaced by summers and winters and geographical locations. Each time different because of the companions I had previously while walking those streets. I can barely remember or recall the senses I had had when viewing the streets years earlier, my whole change in psyche, I mean. Yet there's still a slight trace of what I felt left, a trace filled with the unconcerned dreams and tragedies and longings that make up thoughts before the seriousness of age sets in.

Later, after dark, down at the river, a man emerged from the darkness and sounds of the waterfront, waves turning slightly, raising sounds beneath the wheels of the highway traffic. The guy was large, a strapping laborer's or weight lifter's frame, his hair cropped close to his skull, growing in recently from having been shaved.

I turned on my heel with no hesitation; he turned down by the brick wall that bordered the walkway leading to the crushed sides of the covered pier. Hesitating he muttered something that sounded like a cross between a low whistle and a statement. I followed him as he turned the brick corner and disappeared in the direction of the warehouse. Stepping over rigging irons and broken pipes I followed his retreating back, covered by a black leather jacket that shone softly in the darkness, like shining shoes beneath a surface of water. Stooping beneath the half-raised doorway (loading doors) I saw him walk further into the darkness and then turn suddenly and squat down, motioning me towards him with a single wave of his large hands. Rubbing my palms around the base of his neck over and over, feeling the bristle of his shaved skull against the sensitive undersides of my wrists, movements like birds in a stationary flexing of wings, my hands riding his forehead, smoothing along his jacket, over his hard shoulders and muscles . . . feeling something soft and foreign, I realized he had a couple large feathers hanging from one shoulder by a piece of string, some decoration that perplexed yet gladdened me for it threw meaning into his image, as if it were a tribal gift, a sense of mysterious beauty placed within the projections I had put upon his sturdy shoulders of who he was and what distances he had traveled. His face buried itself beneath my shirt and rose upwards like an enormous fisted hand, tongue easing out between slightly parted lips so I could feel the coolness of a breeze follow his motions. I freed the buckle on my belt and then the button of my overalls, and he followed up with a series of movements of his hands, sliding the zipper down and his face leaning first back and then forward into my belly. I wrapped my hands around his body, my arms pressing against his sides, the wind moving closer and the lights of turning cars spreading beneath the slight cracks in the wall where it joined the concrete floor.

Somewhere behind us in the darkness, men stood around. I could hear the shuffle of their feet, the sense of their hearts palpitating in the coolness, the drift of a slightly luminous hand curving an arc against the night with a cigarette, adrift like falling stars or comets in old comic-book adventure illustrations, a sense of unalterable chance and change, something outside the flow of regularity: streets, job routines, sleepless nights on solitary damp mattresses, a river flowing like a gray film of life past our eyes endlessly, unaltered but by physical actions.

When I came he stood up and whipped out a white rag from his pocket and smoothed it over his forehead and mouth and laughed: Jesus, and I said, Yeah, whew. And he said, The fire really took this place apart, but man if those floorboards could talk . . .

Yeah if those floorboards could talk, if those streets could talk, if the whole huge path this body has traveled—roads, motel rooms, hillsides, cliffs, subways, rivers, planes, tracks—if any of them could speak, what would they remember most about me? What motions would they unravel within their words, or would they turn away faceless like the turn of this whole river and waterfront street, all of its people, its wanderers, its silences beneath the wheels of traffic and industry and sleep, would it turn away speechless like faces in dreams, in warehouses, pale wordless faces containing whole histories and geographies and adventures?

Effects of crashing: It's like you've been bone-tired for the last twenty years and just now suddenly becoming aware of that weariness, the heaviness of it contained within a gesture of a hand, of a gait, or of the turning of vision towards darker things, hoping for eventual and smooth sleep, turning one's back to the shape of the world, looking for rest and respite.

Out along the waterfront asphalt strip, more cars are turning and circling. Headlights like lighthouse beacons drift over the surface of the river, swinging around and illuminating men, strangers, men I might or might not have known because their faces were invisible, just disks of black silhouette outlined briefly as each car passes, one after the other, pale interior faces turned against the windows, then fading into distance.

[No date]

Standing here seeing the outline of my form thrown three times against the glass and metal walls of the doorway, I'm inside, having retreated from the rain. Rain streaking through the spheres of lampposts, making the sidewalks and streets and especially the curbsides boil and foam while taxis sail through it all. One A.M. on the corner of Sheridan Square—across from the unlit triangle of park benches streaming in the night, neons as far as you can see, then the shell of darkness beyond, and back there over that indiscernible line drawn by lack of lights is the whole pocket of memory and a sense of the past few hours, past days, seeds of weariness brought on by the crashings of black beauties.

Afternoon brings me down to the river, a lazy afternoon with the highway traffic rushing along past me, bringing with it all concerns of the working world, schedules blown away in that traffic, in the breeze from the river as I pass beneath the West Side Highway in between slow-moving columns of cars . . .

Inside in one of the back ground-floor rooms of the warehouse, there's a couple of small offices built into a garagelike space. Papers from old shipping lines scattered like bomb blasts among wrecked pieces of furniture, three-legged desks, a Naugahyde couch of mint green upside down, small rectangles of light and river and wind over on the far wall. Met this French guy, born in Paris, working in Los Angeles, has this navy blue sweater with buttons that line the left shoulder, allowing me to slowly fumble in shy awkwardness to set them free, lift my pale hands beneath the sweater, finding the lip edge of his tight white T-shirt, feeling the graceful yet hard curve of his abdomen, his chest rolling slightly in pleasure.

We're moving back and forth within the tiny cubicle, an old soggy couch useless on its side, the carpet beneath our shifting feet revealing our steps with slight pools of water. We're moving around, shifting into positions that allow us to bend and sway and lean forward into each other, arms moving so our tongues can meet with nothing more than a shy hesitation, sunlight burning through the river window empty of glass but covered with a screen that reduces shapes and colors into tiny dots like a film directed by Seurat. His mouth parts, showing brilliant white teeth within the tan of his face, hands unhooking the buttons at the front of my trousers, the arc of his back sending indiscernible shivers through my arms and legs—haunted by the lines of shadows that dip down around his warm neckline, I lean down and find the collar of his sweater and draw it back and away from the nape of his neck and gently probe it with the tip of my tongue.

Later he took me back to his place belonging to a friend of his who is on retreat, and in the shadows of the living room he pulled a gleaming new guitar from its case and proudly rubbed his hands along its neck. We rolled some weed and he made toast and tea and upstairs in the bedroom we got it on again and he fell back into a relaxed state, his arms outstretched and eyelids closed down, his body brown from some faraway sun, and I let one hand slowly explore him, touching, sliding gently over every inch of surface, dipping around the legs, between them, up the hips, following the lines of muscles, the curve of his limbs, the collarbone, fingers smoothing out his forehead, brushing his temples, dreaming whole relationships against his reposing body.

He told me he lived in the States for five years, at first with a boy his own age who was heavily into drugs. The police were after him so they moved in silence to Jersey near where I was born along the sea, and he worked and supported both of them, the other being unable to work for fear of discovery. After two years he left him because of differences that threatened to drive him crazy. The other guy was into S/M: I would beat him up not because I had any desire to, or that I felt anything sexual, but because he wanted it and I wanted to give him pleasure. He finally committed himself to a mental hospital and all the doctors said the same thing: Stop seeing this guy.

And now, two years later, I still miss him . . .

Now it's the next day, having taken some amphetamines yesterday, staying up all night working with clay and paint to produce a yellow-spotted black salamander.

Came into the city and called this Frenchman. He said, Come on over, and I walked through the streets with a sense of weariness, drinking from a clear glass bottle of seltzer water, feeling heat from thoughts and the drift of images from the day before. Realizing his handsomeness and wonderfully outgoing nature was composed of honesty with himself and trusting his senses. He put it forth so clearly while in the presence of a stranger.

We dropped some quaaludes and went upstairs into the bedroom.

Time's become strange, with the distance growing between me and Brian. There's moments when I wish I had some money and a fast car so I could step out the door and burn rubber through gravel and create a separation in my head from the past. Sometime I want to say it to him, to tell him I understand what he's doing. And yet there's this mixture of an emotional *slap* I feel, it's like he's dragging it out on me. Why doesn't he just split and be honest about it, rather than let it die so slow? That's when I wish I had the car. The car and the money to leave this state behind, to leave him behind, so that these senses could slowly fade and eventually become relegated to the past fold of memory, where things assume that drift of function, that drift which allows a cool distance, a view, that emits no color to flush the cheeks.

Los Angeles for a couple days was like some kind of refuge—from the thoughts about Paris and the constant limbo I feel I'm in by allowing fears of the unknown—aging—to keep me standing on all this solid ground. Solid ground, composed of no movements that suggest chance or change from what's momentarily comfortable or safe. I gotta break away from this. I gotta try to take apart and rearrange and step away from this past, step into what could possibly be a new shift in my living.

Sitting in Gary's place: seeing all these little things from Brian to him. They're like Xerox copies of tenderness, the small things that comprised Brian's actions that I took as some kind of symbols of what he felt for me in a *personal* way. Seeing replicas of those actions makes them no longer personal. I feel foolish, like placing dreams in someone else's hands. So this is what it feels like, staring awkwardly across a table, cigarettes in hand, creating a slow haze across little notes in semi-French, a truck of yellow-brown plastic that dispenses Pez candies. Notes that no longer show up on the table at home. Why am I so silly about all this? Being sentimental is okay but when it occurs for lack of real emotions it sucks and seems pointless. Brian asks if I want to do the big "H" tonight. I don't know. Maybe. If the Frenchman doesn't show up in time to change my mind. The thing that makes me feel silent and brooding with the Frenchman is the realization that all this is my background, a whole group of desperate people, while all I really want to do is be feeling excited by living and possibility and desire. Not to nullify it with pills and needles.

There's never been a more foreign kind of rest than heroin, sweet white heat that enters the body slowly (unless it's booted with that slight drawback of blood, then the plunger of the needle pressing fast). A white heat that brings on a sensation of heaviness, of strange weight to the arms, legs, and torso, up around the base of the neck, warmth, and the continual sensation of these weighted limbs immersed in warm fluids, pools of water, lying down with the head slightly raised. A pleasure.

Gary and Val went for the stuff somewhere on 8th Avenue around Times Square, left in a taxi while I stayed behind to wait for Viola who'd broken a bone in her hand just the previous day after catching it in a door. Later in a slight midnight rain as Val and I walked down 8th Avenue to the West Village he told me, God, here I was standing outside this fuckin' restaurant, see, it's a fuckin' front for this dealer, and I wasn't allowed up, so I'm standin' there in my leather jacket and this guy comes up out of nowhere, all these fuckin' hookers paradin' around, right? And this guy comes up and says, Hey, ya wanna go with me for a drink? And I says, No thanks, sweetheart. Then this other guy comes up and starts askin' me if I know where the Barnum Room is, some transvestite disco club, so I thought, Oh gawd, what if my parents ever saw me right here leaning against this bogus facade of a restaurant, fuckin' nighttime in Times Square waiting for a friend who's scoring some heroin . . .

They all showed up sometime later. It was a sublet joint Gary was stayin' in on the fringes of Chelsea, not too far from the apartment of a guy whose head I almost bashed in when I lived on the streets 'cause of his

American Indian stonework collection, this twenty-pound stone fish, black rock, that I wanted as soon as I touched it. Viola walks in and says, Oh gawd, I'm in pain, where's the fuckin heroin? She reaches into her shoulder bag and pulls out a fistful of hypos. Now I gotta find one that works . . .

She's popping the plastic tops off and dipping them one by one into a glass of water, testing them, and finally selects one and pulls the depressor out of the hypo and dips it in a jar of Vaseline, rolls it slightly and sticks it back in. Asks Gary for a spoon: These designer spoons, the guy who sublet this place will kill me if he finds 'em bent. The spoon's bent and the smack is taken out of the tiny snap-lock bag and unfolded from its wrapping. Who's first? asks Viola. Can I be first? She's gonna shoot half of a fifty-dollar cut. Gary and Val say, No, you better do David first 'cause once the needle's out of your arm you'll prolly be in no shape to do anything but nod. So I sit down as she cuts off a quarter of the hit and pushes it onto a matchbook cover and drops it into the bent spoon, a red candle nearby flickers and she's singeing arm hairs, cooks it and drops a wad of cotton from a Q-tip into the spoon and draws the liquid into the needle through the cotton. My arm is tensed up with a robe belt around the biceps and they're both marveling over them big fuckin' veins. Always said I'd make a good junkie. Put your arm down and hold still, she says, a fuckin' pro. The needle slides in easy but she don't boot it since it's my first time. I remember when I was shootin' the coke at her place, her sister the nurse said, Don't worry, if ya drop dead we'll just toss ya outta the window. The plunger pushed and it slides out. Now hold your arm up and rub it so you don't get an air bubble. A minute later I look and can't even find a needle mark. No red dots, nothin'. That's how good she is, Sister Roxanne, nurse of the Netherworlds. Walked over to the couch and lay down and returned to reading the sleazy b-mags the people that own this place left behind: *National Enquirer* and *Star,* etc. "I was Elvis's secret lover for fifteen years." "Tree leaps off hillside and attacks the car of drunken driver." Etc. Waitin' for the effects to come on, feelin' impatient, finally it does, real slow while Viola's takin' the needle from her arm going, Aahhh shit, what a fuckin' rush, having booted it.

Finally it came on and I stopped readin' the mags, swept them off the bed and lay back, oh yeah, oh yeah, and lay there feeling warm and not wanting to budge. Television on in the corner with no sound. Later Viola shuffles out the door trying to figure an excuse to get outta work but heading there nonetheless for night duty. Gary leans across the bed and kisses me good-bye first time, I loved him for that gesture though I couldn't move and conversation seemed silly so I stayed silent. Val and I sitting there for a while then getting our coats on and leaving, walking downtown in the rain, a quick bite at Tiffany's restaurant on Fourth Street and down into Soho via Italian neighborhoods, all-night bars, neon in the drizzle, we're talking friendly and I'm feeling mellow and I say, I feel like I've really lost my innocence, now that I finally have fucked with needles, the whole romantic attachment to them being blown with the first shot. Now it's just down to the simple level of intake and warmth. Whatya mean? he says. You think we'd be walkin' in this fuckin' rain talkin' like this if we'd lost our innocence? And he was right. We walked through Chinatown checkin' out kung-fu movie posters and over into his old neighborhood where we caught the train, shook out our wet jackets, and made it home.

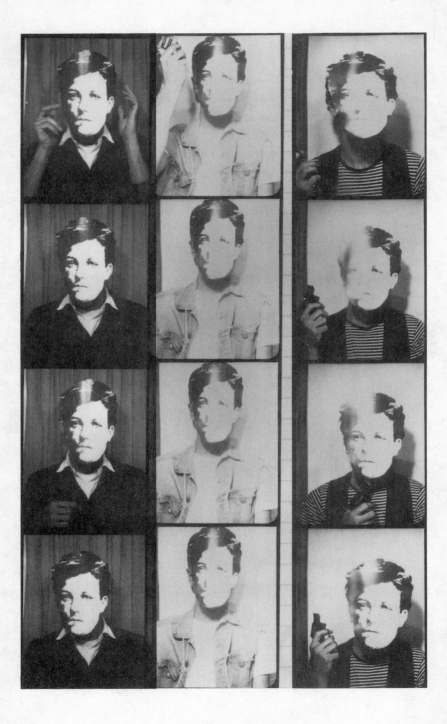

In the spring of 1980, David sent his Rimbaud series of photographs, "Arthur Rimbaud in New York," 1978–79, to Soho News, *a local weekly that covered the art world and downtown scene at the time. Its publication significantly affected his ability to see himself as a visual artist. That same year, his work appeared in three group shows in Lower Manhattan.*

May–June 1980

May 11, 1980

Julius Bar, 7:00–7:30 P.M. Standing around in Julius Bar. Minutes earlier I had run into Jim. He asked me why I hadn't come to Danceteria last night. John had me down on the guest list but I had felt this ache in my stomach probably from the past few days of nervousness because of the *SoHo News* photo deal: the continual delay of definite answer as to whether they planned to use the Rimbaud series or not. So I told him why I hadn't come but mentioned that I was interested in working for him. He said the only stuff available was the same job John was doing. I said fine, and he said to call him Tuesday night. He introduced me to a guy named Riccio, a stage manager for Danceteria. I was so nervous and elated at getting the job I almost fell over a chair on my way out. So I call John, hip him to the news, and fall into Julius, some interesting characters hanging out in the dark open doorway, sounds of conversation floating out, clinking of glasses, jukebox music, etc. I make my way over to the counter and order a beer and the bartender slaps this cool wet bottle on the counter and I make my way with it back to the door. Standing there for some minutes drinking from it slowly, watching this character looking like one of the guys in a Jean Genet prison movie scene with low white T-shirt over powerful hairy chest. My eyes follow down to his stomach packed tight beneath the shirt, down his legs to his highly polished black leather shoes, thinking I've seen this all before, feeling a bit weary suddenly, and my beer is half finished and all the chattering in the bar is getting louder in waves like when you have a fever, I'm thinking suddenly about leaving, eventually turning towards the door, the streets out there leading to other scenes, people, sounds, and occurrences. As I'm turning towards the door, this guy walks up, turns the corner of the street and moves up to the door. I have a sudden snap of recognition—a different quality—something in that stranger tells me he's either transient or different in terms of his sensibilities. I feel something not usual about him, not routine in my daily revolution of faces and personalities and leanings. He steps up into the noisy darkness of the bar, moves slow into the crowded space, steps past and moves over to the counter, hands buried deep in his pockets, hair unruly and sweeping back over his ears, brown lovely hair, strong face, a look around his temples and eyes, a gaze that suggests real thinking and other concerns. I'm taking swigs from my bottle, tapping time, feeling a sense of myself there and nowhere else, not my usual drift where I'm standing silent in a bar in my head moving through other places in the city or the world. Our eyes met a number of times. I remember looking away when the gaze reached a point when it was obvious and strong, turning away to deal with that, feel it through and make some kind of sense of what was coming up inside. Then suddenly he walked up to me and spoke. We talked loosely for a few minutes and I learned he was a filmmaker. I told him of my thoughts about doing a film in Super-8. He was all for it—working with Super-8—said that's how he started.

What followed is difficult to write about, as it's difficult to write about most things that affect me in such a way as to rearrange my view of the world and the lines my life follows within it. But it was beautiful and amazing. We walked in various directions finally ending up by the river. Somewhere out on the docks he turned towards me and embraced me and we made love out there. Later, sitting by the side of the river, he kept leaning over while talking and staring into my eyes. He slipped his hand into mine and my reaction to that was almost bewilderment insofar as people rarely do that in this city, much less when they hardly know you, and I really dug it. A defenseless warmth. We made plans to get together in a couple days, and we left each other after an embrace on the corner of Christopher and Hudson Streets. After walking half a block I turned to look back, and he was standing there, hand in pocket, the other hand up waving. I waved back and turned towards the subway and home.

[No date]

Walking off the curb on 10th Street and 7th Avenue I ran into Arthur. He was making his way towards Julius Bar where we'd agreed to meet. I was remembering him from the other night when I'd met him there, the ensuing walk down into the darkness of the avenues bordering the river, the long stroll out along the broken boards of the pier and the stretch of winds out there, the whole canopy of darkness swelling out from the river's surface and erasing the lines of the dock, the forms of people that moved like silhouettes against the Jersey coast, the removal of ourselves from the rushing city, out there hundreds of yards from the highway and the drag queens and the cruising autos along the asphalt strip, never really having seen his face so clearly as just then bumping into him on the street corner with late sunlight revealing every detail of the street and the characters rushing by him.

We stopped in a dive Greek coffee shop I'd never been in before and had sandwiches and an omelet and afterwards walked down to the river. I was feeling kinda self-conscious, mostly in the aftermath of all those sensations having come up the previous night, of real honesty, of talking and touching, something that at times seems so foreign in this city, times when I start feeling like that communication and contact I have with some characters is what the movements of the world is all about, senses that are really a part of me and my vision of things but haven't much of a place to be expressed. I wanna try and make this more clear—it's like after so many contacts with characters who have lined their bodies and mannerisms and visions with so much guard like gate after gate over solitary rooms, there are these experiences of dealing honestly with people, of laughter and an unguarded movement through living and time and aging, that some of us rarely have a chance to express, rarely feel the freedom to express, rarely feel the freedom to express in the company of others. And so in those moments that previous evening it kind of all opened up at once with him and left me feeling amazed and excited and so here it is a couple days later and I'm wondering what the contact is gonna be like, if the senses will remain real and warm or if a great deal of that was some kind of projection, that kind that some of us put on the forehead of another in unexpected times and moments.

So we hit the pier just as the sun was starting to lose its intensity, and we strolled out towards the end of the dock, couples sitting on the long square timbers lining the edges of the dock, joggers out making the rounds with sweaty bodies and hair drifting and dogs racing back and forth and the waters of the river gliding by nonstop like the unraveling of a film. Arthur was explaining his ideas for this next film he's gonna shoot, these scenes of child abuse: a film of a man making a film on child abuse, in particular, scenes of the kid's exit from his family into the life and arms of the filmmaker, of loving between the filmmaker and this fourteen-year-old kid. Some of his comments: These changes in personality or roles where kids when they're having sex with an older person grow up suddenly, assume postures and manners of an older person, become more serious, whereas the older guy becomes much more like a child. Yet when the scenes are over and they're out on the street, the kid becomes a kid again and the older person resumes the manners and posture of the older person he is. It amazed me, that sense of perception, my flashbacks of the times I'd taken off from home and lived on the streets and the scenes I became involved in, the older men I'd lain down with and the recollection of my movements, my mannerisms with them, those scenes in dim-lit rooms in Jersey swamp motels manipulating a cigarette in my fingers and reflecting on my life and past while talking in a purposefully more sophisticated manner, out loud to the man unseen in the bathroom combing his hair before a fluorescent-lit mirror. A sense of my life at that moment came circling back to me as I lay down there on the hard boards of the dock with the sun turning this strong rose color and slipping so much faster behind a bank of clouds. We lay on our sides facing each other and every so often he reached over and placed a hand on my arm or my leg or my neck and I felt that sense of amazement from the previous night re-newed and the sky and the turning of the earth and river on its axis assumed that quiet and timelessness that comes only in the more peaceful moments when the body is in some state of grace and ideas and thoughts become thor-oughly bound up in the quiet state of the unfolding scenes around me.

This Chinese kid was standing nearby and working with two rods and reels baiting them with large worms and casting them off into the river, and at some point when the sky became more dense and darkness was descending behind the light he caught an eel which he reeled in and unhooked from the line and left tossing on the boards of the dock, the animal's looping dives and thrusts against the rapidly turning blues of the water, reaching for that flow again and again, finally I couldn't stand to see it that way no more and got up and moved over asking the kid if he planned on keeping it. He said no, and I leaned over picking it up and tossed it back in, this iridescent shine left in the palm of my hand which reflected the light of the disappearing sun when I turned it certain ways. There was an intense blue there when I lay back down and turned my face towards the sky, an intense blue with one line of wind-strewn clouds much like northern sunsets I'd seen revolving over Canada from the ridge overlooking the St. Lawrence River, and as Arthur talked, murmuring words that fell across the boards, and later as he started singing, this clear voice unraveling across the river's surface, gently probing the gathering night, I felt this warmth in my belly, a contentedness which had long been foreign. Things got more quiet and the faces of the characters standing, leaning, or lying by the edges of the dock grew more distant and faint and eventually indiscernible. And later we got up and slowly walked back towards the city, the sounds of the traffic like swells on the river, the movements like clockwork overtaking the distance and prolonged time felt way back there by the waters.

[No date]

In the darkness of the room, at various times in the midst of lovemaking, my hand moving through layers of darkness to rest on his chest, on the broad curves of his back, bringing his face close to mine and peering at each other, some words murmured occasionally of how good he felt or how he enjoyed just looking at me, at my being handsome, the spark within his eyes, the sensation of desire in my chest and belly, the relief of being touched and talked to so clearly . . .

He said, You know, I don't think you've been appreciated; you've been loved and bedded and desired, but I don't think anyone's ever appreciated you. There's a sense of sadness about you, a streak of it, something I'm responding to . . .

I was kneeling in the darkness, hands on the ledge of the bed, knees straddling his shoulders feeling this explosive orgasm, the dim light from the courtyard windows easing across the surface of the wall, the sense of his body beneath me, his voice broke through. Put your mouth on mine. I inched back and swung my legs to the side, placed my mouth, my hands on his chest. He put his palm on my chest and raised me away from his face. Now on my cock. And I swung down over him, placed his hard cock in my mouth and immediately he began coming and I heard soft sounds come from his mouth and the darkness in the room moving, stirring with the low breeze over the sill.

He said he was deaf for one year early on in his life. He said, When my hearing returned, I started verbalizing like crazy; I never stopped talking, ever since I've been a verbal person.

[No date]

Met him at Julius Bar last night, standing outside the din of talk and jukebox disco and glass and bottle noise. He rounded the corner in the semidarkness and I crossed the street to meet him. After a brief stop for some food we walked up to 25th Street to his friend's house and made ourselves comfortable on the mattress, which we pulled out of the couch frame. At some point I showed him my photos, the Rimbaud series, and he made comments that I wasn't a still photographer, that I could be doing cinema, moving pictures, because of the evident space in the photos, the sense of them as just a clip from a series of movements, the layout of space in frames was somewhat like an Eastern eye, the middle of some of the photos a blank space. I gave him at his request the self-portrait sunlight photo and a couple Rimbauds: Coney Island and the Longleys restaurant photo. I tried to explain to him the intensity of my feelings since meeting him, and it couldn't really be explained. I don't wanna be like some love-struck kid, though that's okay in itself, just wish I could convey the seriousness of the feelings and the confusion I'm experiencing as an afterthought. Sometimes I wonder if how he sees me is really how I see myself: he sees large streaks of loneliness, etc. At one point reading into my self-portrait he saw loneliness and pain and simultaneous strength and invitation, an extended invitation for the viewer to get to know me.

This sentence came through my head but I realize I would never utter it: I'm not a lonely person, I never feel loneliness. At this point I don't know what loneliness is. In view of the past year and gradually removing myself from most people I knew, I wish I could explain that process, somehow it seems like a catch-22. I slowly removed myself from the company of most people I knew because they were too serious and had laid claim to the whole sense of giving in to seriousness. Most people I knew for the last four years have grown older than their age and laugh little and have grown cynical and tired and see little humor and don't seem to have any energy to really live and experience things fully and richly and that is what I tried removing myself from. But in the process I found myself walking the streets alone most times, being home alone, and gradually falling into a state of very little communication, all because of the desire to preserve my own sense of life and living. So here it is, I've met this guy who feels and talks about things and concerns so very close to my own, but I remain quiet when I want to be unguarded. He talks about fantasies of traveling with me by train or car or hitchhiking, through small towns in the West, through places in this country, and I can't help but respond to them strongly, wishing quietly that it were something other than fantasy, that we were actually going to do these things within a short period of time. He said that in thinking about me he was going to avail himself of those desires, something like air, like water, and that I was the first person since '74 or '76 that he'd met who caused him to consider those things in regards to his movements through this country and this world. He said that I was one of those people that he wouldn't mind seeing turn up anywhere, whether in turning a corner in Amsterdam or in San Francisco or wherever, in turning a corner and seeing me turn a corner in his direction simultaneously, that it would make him very happy. And the sense of those words washing over me while I was lying there on my back in the dim light, my hand stroking out patterns against the hair of his chest, of his arms . . . I wish there were some method of conveying these senses to him, senses that simultaneously make me feel very good and unnerve me because of the probably transient makeup of our contact and friendship. I guess what I'm feeling is that this isn't going to last and that there are very rare times in my life when I've connected with someone who has these sensibilities and articulate language that both excite me, stimulate me in a creative and living sense, as well as confirm senses of my own that lie dormant for long periods of time, that point one can get to where one wonders if the desires one has have any place in the environment, like if I'll ever have a chance to explore these senses in words, in communication with someone who won't be perplexed or who won't deny their realness.

May 27, 1980

Worked this joint (Danceteria) my first weekend. Amazing! A fucking dive, too. Got a job through Jim as a busboy carrying cases of beer back and forth up and down stairs keeping the bartenders supplied with iced Heineken and Budweiser transporting broken sacks of ice to other floors and diving into the human walls of sweating pounding thrusting dancing bodies to sweep up broken bottles and retrieve those about to be broken. Emptying garbage cans mopping bathroom floors and dance floors as each bottle breaks or as drinks are dropped pulling bottles and whole rolls of paper towels out of toilets, etc., etc., etc.

Gives me this strange perspective on New Wave characters. Previously have gone to clubs and just enjoyed myself. But to clean up after these people is another story. Suddenly New Wave is boring and repetitive and predictable. As Arthur said, These people are really like strict conservatives practicing their idea of what it is to have freedom. No imagination. Limited as they are, freedom can only be exercised with destructive actions. They think destructiveness is anarchy. Given a window and told they can do whatever they want with it they would more often break it. There's no imagination in that. How is it really anarchistic? An anarchist would probably say, What window? An artist or someone with imagination would at least paint or draw on it. Mutants were okay, nothing more. I wasn't thrilled by their music. Ended up bored and exhausted but made 100 bucks and 20 dollars tips from the bartenders.

Second weekend it got real bizarre. Some interesting characters but the sweat and toil of the work throws a bizarre slant onto any appreciation. One girl who worked there did smack and fell out on the staircase moments after the joint opened. Apparently a lot of people there are into heroin. I smoked reefer with her day before (Friday night).

Have been spending time on and off with Arthur. I really don't understand what it is I feel for him any longer. I had some pretty strong feelings in regards to him, but that's cooled down in the face of the realization that this whole contact is like passing strangers. Can't escape the sensation at times that I'm just filling out his days till he leaves for Amsterdam. (Today's his birthday, May 27th, and his "angels" have come through with the bucks to finance his next film. Angels being a couple of doctors he knows. Am glad for him.) When we talk, rather when I talk seriously, he gets this drift in his eye like he's in other places. I don't think I'll ever understand the purpose of his telling me that second night on the pier about his having a lot of love to give but others he directs it towards are afraid to return it. For he remains a very private person to me. I feel like I've hardly touched the surface of his sensibilities, he's never broached the subject of what it is he feels about me in terms of time. We only seem to get together and make love— lie down with each other and very little is said. Other than sexual comments or romantic stuff which is fulfilling in only a certain sense. I try to understand it; I realize I don't especially want him to profess undying love to me or commitment of lifelong nature. But I also don't want to remain so uncertain of what it is he feels about me. Of course there's the fear of being liked only for the sexual part of our contact. I'd rather be alone, rather be back in that solitary space walking the streets and viewing the city and the world from a moving vantage point than anchor down sexually and open up these here confusions and longings and heightened verbal senses and then have to pack it all up again in a couple weeks' time. I'm also still very much in love with Jean-Pierre, in a sense that I still desire him in Paris. Jean-Pierre was the first man I was with who was unafraid of my personality or my creative movements. There was room with him to love and live and grow and change. Time has put a distance between us. And my meeting Arthur filled up that kind of empty space. Haven't gone to the piers to get it on with people for two weeks. Connection with Arthur has some intensely great parts and then some real low points: time he has for me, his lack of real attention towards me when I speak, slight edge of impatience until he's talking about his own concerns. So he's turned forty, I think, maybe more, maybe less. I sometimes wonder if he realizes his perspective will surely be vastly different from mine. Once he told me I was naïve in something I said. I agreed. But I think at times he needs someone either unquestioning/young/vulnerable/etc. or someone right on a par with his vision of things. Anything outside of the two might not do in regards to a lover.

So I continue to write to J.P. and I wish I could be leaving to go there soon. And then there's the tension of this contact with Art and also with just recently doing things with my creative work. It gets tense at times. I want J.P. and Paris and a cooling out from the demands of this particular city, and yet I want to do things here rather than feel I'm running away from difficult scenes. I've felt confused a lot since meeting Arthur. It's good in one way in that I have to examine my desires and goals and ideas from everything like possibly living with J.P. and what it is I want to do while I'm here. At times though I wonder if I will ever meet someone who will thoroughly replace my love for Jean-Pierre. That's always been a somewhat scary thought as I would hate to be in a position of suddenly not feeling that love any longer. When I think back to Paris and Touquet and quiet times in that tiny eight-by-twelve-foot courtyard room with the window-sill as our refrigerator, I get such intense feelings of longing to be able to share J.P.'s life again. When I met Arthur he awakened some dormant senses in me. Things I've wanted to feel and experience and communicate freely for so long. There was a fear and tension there for a while that I would slowly draw away from J.P. towards Arthur. But so much is lacking in the contact that I guess I no longer have to fear that. And what is lacking seems to be almost indefinable. That's what is strange and hard to understand.

Anyway, now I'm almost done writing a film script for a black-and-white silent film, thirty to sixty minutes in length. Arthur plans to lend me his old Super-8 to film it with. Friends have offered to play parts in it. Spent the morning at home typing the shots out, and am incredibly dazed from the silence of home, the intense cigarette smoking during the writing, also a lot of tension coming up in realizing how difficult some of these scenes will be to film and the simultaneous desire to get those scenes filmed despite cost or difficulty or even impossibility in regards to finding a guy to play the main part.

Dennis almost got murdered by some demented guy on the bridge a week or so ago. Talked to him last night. Upset me to hear this. Death coming so close to myself, to people I have shared part of life with. Sucks. Thought of years ago on the streets having come close to being killed myself by that madman posing as a cop down by the buses parked on 40th and 11th Avenue.* How it was at that time and age, the closeness of death dispelled by the relief of having been able to escape it. Now years later I feel our mortality more. Being in my midtwenties I sense the completeness that an unexpected death would be. I fear death and disablement, I feel the fear and horror of death coming close to friends. And I remember Lee's brutal murder in uptown hallway when I was nineteen or twenty.

June 18, 1980

Hey Alex:

How r u? Got your letter a couple days back. Great photos, them windows, thanks for passing them on. Just got up this morning at some semistranger's house up on East 16th. Warm house fifteen stories up with little balcony outside filled with vegetables and flowers growing. Sun coming up it was about 5 A.M. and the cool colors of the foliage and trees and vines and ivy and corn and snapdragons and tomatoes and jungle plants all flowing out from cool shadows into the light—special morning this. Felt pretty good knowing the *SoHo News* was out and waiting round the corner for me to check it out. Scary sensation of, Oh shit is it gonna look silly or what? This guy I was staying with last night was someone I ran into recently who is gonna make a motorcycle trip across the United States in another month

*David describes this story in a monologue, "Boy in a Coffee Shop on Third Avenue," in *The Waterfront Journals*.

and that's got me frazzled like Jesus here it is after such a long time wander-
lust has hit me smack in the face again and all week long image after image
in books in film in memories turning over and over in the skies unfolding
behind river dusks, images of past travels and images of possible travels, all
these sensations having lain dormant for some time now have suddenly
emerged again and I'm starting to feel a bit alive again. The last so many
months have been like ether to me what with dullness spreading and feeling somewhat alienated in who and what I am in regards to others. My God,
listen, in the issue of *SoHo News* there's an article on Jayne Anne Phillips
and in that very article are things/statements she makes that for the first time
in my life, in my recent years, articulate exactly what I've been feeling. What
flips me out is that great fuckin' realization that it's not just me. You don't
know how much better that makes me feel. So anyway there's a slight chance
that I might accompany this guy, what it will take is just cuttin' the strings
to New York and that furious dog of security and then I can be on my way.
Dunno for sure if it'll come off or if this stranger will go buzzin' off in westerly
directions by himself. But despite that I still got the urge and if it's what I
should do I can find ways to do it.

After I left the apartment, I picked up the copy of the paper and walked
for ten blocks through East Village before I had the nerve to open it to first
page and was instantly delighted at the fact they gave me extra exposure on
page one, yeah! Walked another five blocks before I had guts to open it to
centerfold, how silly I can be. And yeah yeah yeah, really think it looks
good, am so fuckin' pleased with how they handled the layout. I had asked
them for that repeat of photos of Rimbaud wounded, but the text was done
so much better in terms of different sizes of type. Lookin' at the whole page
is great. There's just so much going on in there, so much info visual and
word. Whew . . .

So Danceteria is opening an extra night a week, you and Lois have to
come down one night, I'll call ya soon and we'll set a date for it and I'll put
you on the guest list, okay? I'm supposed to see the Picasso show (Pablo
Picasso was never called an asshole) in July. The upstate parties were good
especially the car scenes on return as I've taken photos of friends sleeping
but always wanted one of myself in that state, totally unconscious, ya know?

Last Saturday night at Danceteria was the worst ever. Now I'm head busboy and run all three floors helping the other busboys out. Chuck, this great guy who usually gets stuck with the main floor and is now a good friend, we was runnin' nuts with the crowd breaking stuff up and dropping bottles like those newsreels of bombs floating out the bottoms of airplanes. A pipe in the wimmen's room burst twice sending cascades of water everywhere. You don't know what tough means till ya stepped into a crowd of wimmen in a tiny john in a rock club at 3 A.M. with mops and alla them turn around and abuse ya while yer tryin' ta mop the fuckin' floods up and some woman's doing Chaplinesque stumbles with a beer in one hand and a head fulla quaaludes and sayin' does the bus stop here? Then later we found her in the men's room calmly discussing an elephant-sized turd draped over the top of the only toilet. We said, Fuck this, man, the salary ain't that good, and left the rest of the desperate Danceteria boys to deal with it. Then at some point when we both were gonna quit for the twentieth time, Chuck spied these two assholes on the main dance floor throwing each other about the floor, "artfully arranging themselves into living sculptures," and ran over and kicked the guy square in the ass and said, Git up muthafucka (he's from Memphis) you ain't the only person in this joint, and left the guy yellin' at the top of his hack daniels lungs, He KICKED me he *kicked* me. Jesus gimme a break . . .

Brian's been ill. Lady Doc told him yesterday he may be the first person in twenty-five years to have rheumatic fever. Test comes back today and we'll find out thank god it ain't contagious.

So this has been my life this past week. Oh yeah, Carole (remember her from Bookies) appeared before me at Danceteria like a vision in leather jacket and crow black hair askin' for a Heineken. Had a good long talk and we'll get together sometime in the near future. She's movin' into town in two weeks.

Look, I'm light-headed from no food since last night, gotta run and buy somethin' to eat before my ears fall off. Good to get yer letters, hope all is well and hello to Lois and Mike and Mona and we gotta get together soon okay? Bye-bye.

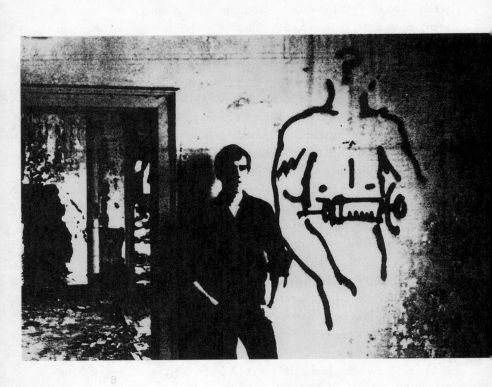

[No date]

Down in the piers going towards sunset, the river easing into dusk, times I think I see myself from a distance entering the ribbed garagelike doors of this place from the highway, times I gain a certain distance from myself and wonder why it is these motions are continued, animal sexual energy, the smell of shit and piss becoming overwhelming insofar as everyone uses this joint as an outdoor toilet, getting fucked and letting it loose in some spare corner, rage from months of old sex, stained clothes, and pools of urine. To get past this you have to breathe light and stay near the openings of the walls and walk way back to the end where the walls open out into the river and some concrete platform that rides out a ways and every so often crumbles into the sea. Deep in the back of the mind some of us wish it would all burn down, burn away in some raging torrent of wind and flames, pier walks collapsing and hissing into the waters, somehow setting us all free from past histories of this warehouse, of its once long ago beautiful rooms that permitted live films of Genet and Burroughs to unwind with a stationary kind of silence, something punctuated by breathing alone, and the rustle of shirts and pants sliding, being unbuttoned or folded back. Walking towards the entrance, the sun had gone down behind the Jersey factories leaving just a pale darkness inside the place, figures could appear and disappear, become vacant or nonexistent. Suddenly out of one of the side rooms that once had been a loading dock there was a series of high-pitched hysterical screams and in all of that gathered darkness a figure of light flew out, speed motions of arms and legs pumping, propelling it towards the far wall, blur lines of movement, an abject silence following in the wake of screams, and I immediately thought to myself: stupid queen. For there were times in the past when drag queens, weary of the lonesomeness amidst all this blatant standing in doorways, made clinical comments on the muffled sounds of interlocked limbs. But this time the figure stood in dim light holding one hand to his neck and shaking. Several guys and myself rushed over.

There's a guy in there with a knife. He cut me, he said, turning his head to the side, exposing a long red wound on pale white skin. I turned blindly, rushed along the floor till I found a door that had been ripped off its hinges, and tugged like a madman at a two-by-four that had been nailed into its surface: a great roar as the nails pulled out. I rushed with it into the side room looking for the man. The kid had described him: black hair, white guy, mechanic's overalls and blue windbreaker. He said, I thought something was strange about him, like he didn't seem too interested in getting it on, at least not near other people. I had second thoughts, but unfortunately I was too attracted to listen to them. I felt him cut me, and I pushed him away and started running and screaming. There are several small enclosures in the loading dock area; some guy poked his hand through the windows and flicked a lighter while I covered the doorways ready to bash the guy's head if he came running out.

[No date]

Things change when the air changes: that's a statement uttered by some homeless Joe a long time ago, almost a year, when Brian and I first moved into Vinegar Hill. So here it is, I'm sitting in an apartment on 2nd Avenue in the East Village. Second night I've slept here. There's a dog that pisses on everything and tears apart the faded couch cushions and digs to China through the soft stuffing sitting in a chair opposite me watching the clockwork characters' movements, tiny and unattainable on the cobblestone streets below. First time in years when everything is up in the air. I'm unsure of work and it seems a lot of people's lives are on the line, all of them either sleeping or waking across the city right now. The Club was busted last Saturday night. I was coming up from the basement with two water pitchers in my hand. George, the jerk who stands at the exit door, wasn't there. I remember feeling perplexed and wondering where the fuck he'd gone.

Looked around the crowded main floor as I stepped through the door, I caught sight of him as he skulked away with a wounded animal look on his stupid face. He looked right at me but kept on walking. As I crossed the floor with the empty pitchers in my hand to the main floor bar Carol Black ran by right behind me, grabbed me by the shoulder, and said, Cops are here! and continued on. I shook off that image, thinking it was just like the firemen's visit, they'd look around and then split. As I reached the main floor bar, I saw this big beefy detective in a brown suit and striped tie like Alfred Hitchcock standing behind the bar. Behind him, Barbara had a worried look on her face. I reached for the water/mixer hose and a fat cop snapped, Bar's closed! I gave him a disgusted look, waved him away and reached over, grabbed the spigot, and started filling the pitchers. He slammed my hand away and yelled something unintelligible, and I backed away in confusion. Something was happening. I walked around towards the front ticket booth and saw Michael Parker and Lolo and about seven others shoved into the ticket booth illuminated in all that darkness of the hall with fluorescent lights. Others were along the wall. Dick was rushing around. I turned and rushed downstairs, people still dancing and DJ's putting on records like normal. Went over to the bar where Max Blagg and Tim were and leaned over the bar and said, Tim, there's something really weird going on upstairs. Call Max over. Max! There's something going on upstairs. The cops are here, and they got all these people lined up behind the ticket booth with their hands in the air. No sooner had I finished than a hand latched onto my shoulder and spun me around. It was some beefy dick and he held me for a second and stared into my eyes. Then he pushed me away and was joined by a second cop. The first one bent low to go under the counter of the bar but banged his head 'cause there was no opening there. He stood back up and the second cop helped him over the counter. He handcuffed Tim and Max. I was shocked and backed up slowly into the crowd, stood back as they led him out and up the stairs. Upstairs Carol Black grabbed onto me and told me to sit down along the wall like one of the customers. It was clear that anyone working there was being arrested. When the cops were arresting Max I remember looking for a fire extinguisher with the thought in mind of firing it on the cops: these fantastic ideas of creating confusion, setting people free. I stood back and watched him and Tim be led up the stairs to the main floor, following minutes later. Tried to push through the confused crowd to the mezzanine in order to see what was happening to Brian and the others up there. But the cops had gone up before me and were in the process of shoving customers down the stairway to clear the upper floor. Wandering around the main floor, customers yelling for drinks: I just bought drink tickets! Cops punching people around, arresting some momentarily, letting them go minutes later if they did not work in the club. Carol Black grabbed me and pulled me to the side: Pretend you're a customer. We sat down on a side bench, my arm around her shoulder, hers around my waist, talking in undertones to try and make sense of the confusion. Finally cops began clearing customers from the club, threatening them with arrest if they stayed behind. We waited until it was no longer safe to stay and slowly walked out in the last lines of the crowd. Saw seven or more people in the front ticket booth under sickening fluorescent light—a couple with faces bloodied—all with hands in the air looking frightened. Lolo looked at us and moved his lips, Leave, leave, nodding towards the exit.

January 21, 1981

Reagan is the president of this country now. What more or less do we need . . .

I haven't moved to put words down in here in ages, going through a time in my life that seems desperate, surreal, awful, and slightly wondrous, all simultaneously. Met a fellow a month or so ago—Peter Hujar—a photographer who in some interesting ways is like a mirror of scenes I'm entering or have entered. When I talk to him or vice versa, it's like seeing senses unravel that are almost the same, separated by social class or money or something like age attitude. I still have hope in my life somehow. He has the same desperate and at times confused outlook but minus that one seed of hope—a kind of hope or desire that could be bogus or real, but nevertheless I have in me and which helps me ignore the difficult things that surround me, or at least lets me see them as transitory with some future point in store that will absolve me of all this searching or desire or confusion.

New York City

September 1, 1981

I'm sitting in the park up on 15th Street, long after the sun's gone down. I'm sitting there in the darkness under some trees on a bench and this seedy red-haired man in a cheap business suit suddenly walks over and slides onto the bench next to me, simultaneously mumbling something. It sounded like, How does an egg come out? He said it quick, fumbled his dirty hands against each other, quick nervous pats to the hair sweeping around the sides of his ears. I was disturbed by the way he moved up and sat down. I'd been looking at this young guy sitting over on a railing: the young guy was watching the two of us, me and this seedy guy, wondering if we were making contact.

I had no patience: What did you say?

Uh . . . how does one come out?

I felt thoroughly disgusted. The guy had some hideous skin rash, greasy temples. He wouldn't look at me, just stared straight ahead as he talked, his hands like two small bird wings, long nails, clattering against one another. I looked at him hard and snapped, I don't know what you're talking about.

He flinched slightly. You don't know what I'm talking about? How does one come out? How does one go about doing what those guys over there are doing (he motioned towards the park hut where in the leafy shadows I could make out the forms of a series of men in various leaning positions). I mean, I never did it before. I don't know how . . . I wish I could find someone to teach me . . .

Don't worry about it. It comes natural . . .

Yeah, but how do you meet someone? How do you approach someone, like how did those guys start to do it?

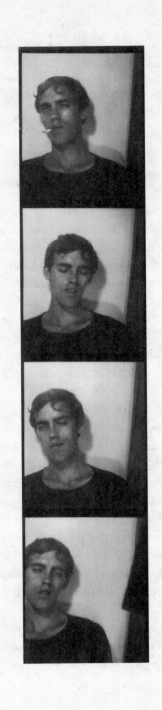

Oh they probably know each other, I said dryly.

He fiddled with his hands some more, and then his voice dropped two octaves, and he said huskily, Uh . . . do you want to get to know me? No.

He sat there for a few minutes staring straight ahead and nodding every couple of seconds like he was digesting the information, then got up and walked away quickly.

I looked towards the railing where the young guy had been sitting and saw that he was talking to some other guy who'd approached him from the pathway. The guy who approached him was large and muscular, handsome in a way, wearing black cowboy boots that clicked as he stepped and shifted back and forth, laughing over some unheard thing, rubbing his hands and then reaching out and putting his hand on the side of the young guy's face, almost caressing it, but the young guy pulled back slightly. A blond man who'd once been overweight and this year had a new body, wearing a tan bodysuit beneath his white trousers, stepped over to me and began with, I know you don't remember me, but we met once before . . .

I got up and started walking, walked around under the lampposts along the Avenue side of the park past a bench where two boys sat, one in the other's arms lying on his back, a slow breeze flowing and the other guy stroking the sides of his head, around the temples, with long white fingers. He said, I wonder what the red sky means. I looked up and the sky had a red pale glow on the bellies of clouds. It was getting towards dawn.

I crossed the street at the center intersection and entered the east park. The regulars were sitting over on the side: these characters take over a few picnic benches and play some sort of card games until all hours of the morning. In the grassy sections of the park behind iron railings were men and women sleeping beneath dark covers.

I went back into the west section and suddenly felt very weary. I hadn't planned on meeting anyone but then I saw this young guy who seemed pretty interesting. He was attractive because he had a complete sense of himself. He was unhurried, sitting back on the rail in the shadows, cool black hair, looking around. I walked over by him, and he looked back at me. I passed him and sat down on a bench nearby, staring at the distances of the park, through the cool leaves, wind, empty benches, and lampposts, losing myself. I wanted to talk to him but felt tired and didn't know if I could handle lying down with anyone. But the idea of walking away and maybe never seeing him again made me stand up, turn slowly in the breeze, and look around at him. He had his head turned but it moved back towards me, and I ended up turning away again, walking a few feet towards the bushes, turning and walking back to the bench, sitting again and standing back up again. I felt absurd, tired, anxious. He kept looking at me. I realized that if I left the park without speaking to him, he might feel I wasn't interested, and at any time after that night if I saw him again he probably wouldn't try to speak with me. I walked past him a second time, felt absurd again, turned back slowly and walked over to him.

How's it going?

Fine, fine, he said smiling. It was one of the most charming smiles I had ever had made towards me. With a flash of white teeth—he was roughly handsome, smooth skin—he reminded me of someone I'd seen in my past, a guy years ago when I was getting on a train somewhere in the dusk of the city, a face among the crowds in the station, someone I never forgot. I sat down next to him, and we talked for a while about the things that we did. He was a photographer. I'd seen some of his things in a weekly paper and one or two books. I felt strange, not from knowing some of his work, but because he was so attractive to me. It wasn't just physical, it was a kind of excitement I felt realizing the distances one has traveled. I listened to his speech; he had a slow grace about him, contained, humorous, no harsh visions of life. His hands, his head and speech moved slowly like he was vaguely stoned but very clear. At some point we left the park and walked down to the Kiev restaurant for coffee. And sitting in the back against the wall we made slow sparse conversation. I knew I wanted to lie down with him but nothing was mentioned. I wondered how it would be approached, if at all. What words, what gestures.

When we left the restaurant I asked him if he was a little stoned and he laughed and said, Everybody asks me that. No. I laughed and apologized, feeling a little embarrassed. I asked him where he lived and he said 12th Street, and I told him I'd walk him part of the way. We headed west down the street glittering with lamps and pools of broken glass, an emptiness in the dark air, a taxi in the distance bouncing over a hole in the street, the sound echoing.

On the way up Broadway we passed the church around 11th Street, which has a front yard with a large urn the size of four men side by side and dark green lawns and some trees and flowers that had recently lost their petals. The entire yard was bathed in night shadows but over the roofs and spires the sky was turning a deep cobalt. I turned to him and said, I haven't lain down on grass in ages . . . We stopped and rested our hands on the wrought-iron fence, white against gleaming black. Then I said, There's too much dog shit in the parks to lay down.

He didn't say anything, but turned and walked over to the gate and reached over touching the latch. It was open. He unhooked it and the gate swung open, and he turned to me and smiled. We stepped inside on the asphalt path and walked along it and then he stepped onto the grass and lay down on his back stretching his arms. I smiled and lay out next to him, the face of the buildings whose yard we were in joined the church, was part of the same architecture but had little shades half-rolled down the windows, some gauzy white curtains, and darkness behind them. I wondered if there were nuns and priests sleeping in well-tucked beds, I thought of clean white sheets, little bed stands with wire-rimmed glasses and handkerchiefs and beads and little plastic saints and angels like those on Avenue D dashboards. We lay there for some slow minutes with our hands beneath our heads staring up: large mobile clouds with reddish tinge to their bellies and the jigsaw sections of turquoise sky behind them, shuttering for moments until they were once again covered, one spire way up catching the gradually warming light of dawn way east of the river and tenements. The yard was still filled with a descending night, like some old Magritte scene. He reached over and touched my arm and I touched back, sliding my hand in between the buttons of his shirt and feeling his smooth belly, muscular and warm. Very warm. He turned on his side half-facing me and I climbed up over him, half on him, nuzzling my mouth against his warm neck, the palm of my hand so perfectly formed to the curve of his head, the soft black hair against my fingers. We kissed as the yard slowly turned light and a bus roared by. I felt very happy quite suddenly, like some chord had been touched, something that I hadn't been aware of needing was just at that moment fulfilled. We lay there in an embrace, not saying anything. It was cool, quiet, the occasional sounds of a faraway city, the wet tips of grass and the warmth of him through his clothes. At some point a couple of bums walked by and I heard one yell, Hey you homos . . . get outta there. We released each other and lay there, one of my arms curved over his chest, and watched the air for a while finally rising from the ground and walking about looking for a place that still contained the night. Nothing. We looked in windows and saw a desk with envelopes and papers on it. He said it was a beautiful garden as we turned around to leave.

He invited me to his apartment and we went there: a small attic studio with two rooms and a kitchen. There was a tree, a small one, or maybe a large branch, nailed to a board on the floor. It was for a photo he was shooting. He said he was going to add a box of fake snow to it. He said he was using some kids in the series of photos but that it was held up because they had all gone to summer camp and wouldn't be returning until the next week. On one wall was a photograph by some French man: a group of male and female children mannequins, in the countryside seated at a picnic bench by a bank of trees, some of the kid mannequins half-rising from the benches with wine bottles in their hands and plates of half-eaten food on the table, and some standing nearby looking dazed by their postures. They were all turned or moving towards an enormous wall of flames not more than ten yards away, trees and hills of the countryside stretched out before them and behind the flames. They all looked drunken, like some scene from Brueghel.

He asked me if I wanted to shower with him and I said yes, and sat down on a nearby couch and began unlacing my ratty sneakers, for a moment embarrassed by them in the dawn light coming from a skylight. He took off his clothes and I was amazed by his tan, a healthy brown band of lighter skin where he had once worn underwear. He turned on the shower and went into another room and I looked at a small photograph of himself in some foreign country on a beach, with a red towel over him, cross-legged, leaning over a book whose one white page he held between his fingers as if in turning, and the sense of him in that photo was even more clear than how I saw him in the park hours before, seated on the railing: that intense sense of completion, of knowing himself and being comfortable with himself, the distances he'd traveled and the life he moved within. Nothing I can really articulate here but it was contained in his posture, his body, his face and fingers.

In the shower I lifted a bar of soap to his back and began rubbing it with handfuls of water over his smooth skin. He turned around finally and did the same to my back, then turned me around so that I faced him and rubbed the soap over my chest and working down to my belly and he raised my hands in the air and smoothed soap beneath my arms in the hair of my armpits down across my belly and beneath my balls, soaping with one hand and smoothing with the other. Then he took some gel from a bottle of shampoo and eased it into my hair, rubbing with the tips of his fingers and it was a sense I hadn't felt since I was a kid, too young to recall, of being vulnerable, of placing my body in another's hands, a sensation that was beyond sex but still very erotic, an emotional sense of relief.

After the shower we made love, and it was a little awkward for me. I wasn't sure of everything, of what movements to make, either because I was weary or because I was overwhelmed. And then we slept. Later, hours later, when we woke up, we made love again and then I pulled on my trousers in a semidazed state. Not enough sleep, some sort of warm delirium from all the coasting images of the previous hours. I had a head full of things I wanted to say but couldn't. I tied my sneakers and left his apartment, walking down the carpeted stairs past curving walls with green printed paper, old and musty but with a sense of unspoken class. Then I was out on the street. It was overcast, which I was grateful for, it felt very easy on the eyes, the city traffic in the afternoon, people standing on street corners, streets filled with cars and buses humming, and even though it was overcast there was some startling nature to the light, everything graphic in detail, a heavy sense of rain in the cool air, and turning a corner to head east and downtown I suddenly smiled, seeing grass stains on my trousers for the first time in years.

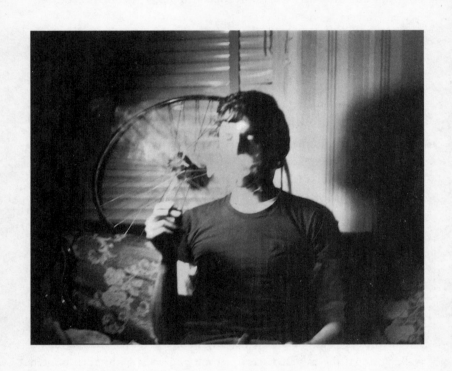

September 21, 1981

After the bust at Danceteria I seemed to have lost trust in any situation or thing. Everything became groundless, apt to fall apart at any moment, nothing offering security or permanence. It wasn't just the arrests or the eventual loss of work, but rather a period of time in which I grew tired of all the scenes I'd been involved with. It shows in a lot of my work: some influences, assimilation of trends or contemporary creative stuff, but at the same time I'm always running from those things, letting my work stem from mostly what affects me in my life, a work composed of impulse and desire to hold particular senses at one time, sometimes embracing them and then discarding them.

Meeting this guy Peter [Hujar]: I was slightly drunk, standing in The Bar on 2nd Avenue, he stared at me and I looked back several times. I guess I wanted him in a strong way, his invitation, a look in the eyes, a feeling of quiet desperation knowing how easily you can hold a person, just wanting that moment to come in time when you have the chance, rather than seeing it slip away in a crowd, glimpsed and then lost. I'd pretty much stopped walking the streets, the coolness of winter and weariness from work in the new club keeping me asleep or lounging and uninterested in walking through the door.

We went back to his place because I had a dog that barked. In his loft he reached into the darkness of a shelf and retrieved a book of his: portraits of life and death or something similar. I knew it, knew it well, and there was that instant where I'm confronted with the enormous image of a person, image gained from previous contact with them, through their work or through pure association with the idea of them in a meeting, like some rogue on the river to whom all the attachments and ideas of Jean Genet I connect, in whom I can place shadows of fiction in the first minute of meeting and speaking, so that this unknown character can assume the air of islands and prison and mystery, something foul and wonderful at the same time, criminal, loner, drifter. And yet the poor guy could be nothing more than a bank employee slumming in the dangerous air of the river, someone with a collection of stone owls at home, with fancy drapes and a Formica kitchen, a new dishwasher, and lace doilies on antique countertops.

So working through this took some time, in the eventual meetings with Peter, in a series of days I let the image of his work dissipate and be replaced with who he seemed to be, his words outlined for himself as himself. Almost a disappointment as always, and yet a relief that I wouldn't be hounded by a head-held image of what I secretly desire in a guy. He actually turned out to be quite human and fallible and because of that, interesting and disturbing. So, he seemed to be going through a series of things that I have been grappling with, but without the hope or sense of living that saves me in my own eyes.

I've showed him much of my work and his response has been one of disinterest or at least of being mostly unaffected by my images. This causes me some sort of extreme discomfort. Last night I left his place after using him in a twenty-second segment of the heroin film that I've been making. I left his place and met later with Jesse and Brian, feeling a lot of anger at the state of my own art, feeling that I'm stuck in some sort of limbo with my work, feeling unencouraged, feeling that I'll never get anywhere with my stuff, as if it is quite meaningless to the people I most want it to have meaning for, feeling that as an artist or person who creates, that I'm basically a failure, that I haven't reached a sort of state that lets creative action be something that has an independent meaning or is capable of affecting change in anyone other than friends. What does this mean? I simultaneously see the absurdity of this, why would I want to effect change, isn't that an impossible desire, isn't change through action? Work, an impossible thing to ask. What is it that I want to change? Maybe I want people to faint at the meaning of my work. What would that be like, fainting through something not like fear or challenge but through a sense of it being so true in this world as an independent existence? This is something I don't think is possible to define. One of the problems is that I dislike the sense of the work I put out, most of it dealing with aggressive images, images that smack people in the face, assault them, or mirror what disturbs them. I seem to really desire some way to seduce people, make them feel at ease and yet make them renounce all the terrible things of the earth and say: Yes, this is what is true. At one time I just wanted to get people to reexamine their ideas of things or get them to experience what they otherwise would not come in contact with, now it's run away by itself and become some intent to change things, which has got to be impossible. I want to be loved for my work, I want people to reel from contact with it, and yet mostly I want them to feel good from it. But the images and scenes I deal with are things of quiet desperation rather than universal beauty, something most people ignore or see as proof of a problematic society or existence.

So now he has called me up and told me that he has syphilis. I've gotten my shot and am in a state of pain and reexamination of all I once held as my life, not because of the shot but because of the weariness of all these daily routines: work, movements, neighborhoods, friends, activities, etc. Also the sense that I'm no longer creating anything, or even further, I'm no longer feeling anything from what I make, wondering if living in a foreign country means any more than continuing to live here, wondering what I could do that would map one's own life in a way that would mean something other than personal reaction, wanting something more universal. But I continue the only ways I know how, always with looking over my shoulder for that chance to change direction and run, escape, depart.

[No date]

Went into the bar on 2nd Avenue after leaving Randy's house. Stopped in for a beer. Just about a dozen or so characters hanging out in there; it was three in the morning. The bartender leaned over and said hello, asked me where I'd been all weekend, and I told him I'd gone away. He gave me my Bud and I stepped back from the bar, and some guy who I hadn't noticed sitting in the line of stools among other people turned towards me and said, Where'd ya go, Minnesota? I could hear the faint edge of sarcasm in his voice, but it was friendly enough all the same so I said, Nope, Maine. He was a guy about my own age, tanned, and his face had some remains of a complexion problem, something maybe in his past as a teenager—sweet looking Joe—reminded me of some gas station attendant, some kid on a summer job from out of state. We joked back and forth and he was obviously drunk, trying to say things and stopping midsentence. I stepped back against the wall and guzzled the beer, first one in four days, and was hit instantly by it. After about ten minutes the blond guy stepped back from his stool, tipping over slightly but managing to find a place along the window next to me. He leaned over and asked some nondescript questions, things like where was I from and some other stuff, still cutting his sentences up every now and then. I found it amusing; he wasn't an unbearable character like most drunks could be, maybe because of his age. He was kind of funny. After a few minutes he asked me if I ever came to this bar to pick up boys and bring them home. I said, Rarely, don't meet many people I'd wanna bring home. He took mock offense at this and said something in return. I told him I didn't drink much and he said he drank a lot, nightly. He was a bartender in some straight joint uptown. I touched his chest and said, Doesn't show though. Well that's because I don't drink beer.

Finally we cut out together and went down along the Bowery towards where he lived. He would give these funny little hop-and-skip jumps into the air, arms up and out like some marionette or person imitating an airplane, several times, almost stumbling to his knees. At one point I said, Gee you sure walk funny, and he smiled and said, Really? Think someone'll notice? This area ain't safe for walking around drunk.

Then he stopped to take a piss behind some Dumpster, in plain view of all the Avenue's traffic. Hey, he said. Is this all right? Nobody can see me, right? Some huge black wino stumbled by and went over to him trying to hit him up for change.

Up at his place, some slightly run-down building that he shared with a bunch of other people, he had his own floor. There were two black kittens racing around. We sat on the couch and started kissing slow-like, touching each other here or there, stopping for a cigarette. He was still drunk but was sobering up a bit from fooling around.

It was almost like a repeat of the guy up in Maine, only more urban, the Bowery alive outside the window with its traffic and muttering winos, inside a house with alley cats chasing each other through the dimly lit room. He was hesitant about getting any further into sex until he finally got up and shut out the lamp, the place went into darkness, just a faint light over the sill coming through the curtains from a streetlamp. We undressed each other and got it on.

After a while I had come and he was having difficulty. He apologized once saying it was from being drunk but I waved it away and said, That's okay, you don't have to come. He said, Yeah, but I want to. Then a second later, Yeah you're right, it ain't necessary. I got up after a while of sitting around on the couch and running my hands along his sides, over his chest and face. Got dressed and sat back down next to him. Ya know, he said (we'd made love all that time still in our socks), I got this fantasy of you and me, it'd be great if we, well, I can just see us in high school together, just coming out of practice or somethin', in the school locker room, boy I'd love to walk in the locker room and see you taking a shower, soaping yourself up all over, just the two of us in there takin' a shower. I was always embarrassed to take showers in front of the other guys in school. Can you do me a favor, please? Can you go over to that chair and start undressing for me? I'd love to see you getting undressed like this was a locker room or something.

I said sure. He was lying back in the darkness on the couch, a faint light from the dawn coming in slow over the windowsill illuminating his brown body, the movement of his arms in this faint blue light as he slowly jerked himself off. I went over to where this chair was in the center of the room and lifted one foot up on it and began slowly undoing my laces. I could feel myself in some faraway locker room, in some dusty scene from my own past and the past of others, urban or country, some makeshift setting, a locale made up of images from novels and from real experiences as he murmured them from his place on the couch. The sound of cries in faraway baseball or football fields, kids in hallways, traffic on faraway streets, blue and pink dusks, and the faded green metal lockers from memories. He gave a small gasp from the vicinity of the couch. He was no longer visible, the dawn light behind the curtains having reduced him to shadows.

[No date]

Sometime in the evening, getting on kind of late. This is a Thursday night. 2nd Avenue full of people, the kinds of people I never really notice anymore when walking down a street, not quite tourists but something like that (characters like middle-aged couples going into Abe's delicatessen or off to see some harmless show), lots of these people, nameless, faceless, almost uninteresting. Something about saying that that makes me feel funny. I always thought anyone could interest me, maybe anyone could, but some nights I hardly even look up from the direction I'm going in to see what I'm passing by. Then again sometimes it's a code of symbols I respond to, a way of gesturing someone has, some criminal element in a stranger's actions that will cause me to look up and notice them. But safe moderate middle-class movements, clothing, speech, and I'll continue walking by without a pause.

I was carrying a book [*Tricks*] by Renaud Camus, some book written by this Parisian about his encounters in different parts of France and America, anonymous encounters with homosexual men. Was bringing it down the Avenue to Peter Hujar's place. He'd photographed this guy when he was in Paris and was interested in reading his book. Peter lives in this loft over on Twelfth and Second, a few flights up.⋆ As I neared the building I could see strobic flashes of light issue from the windows every once in a while. He mentioned he would be photographing Ethyl Eichelberger, a drag queen who writes some wonderful songs and has a lovely voice and performs on an accordion and ten-inch heels, tap-dances, too. I had caught her act up at some club uptown the previous Sunday with Peter. She sang some songs about various lovers, a sailor met in a park, amphetamines, etc.

I got him on the phone from the street below, explained I had the book with me: Hi, Peter. I saw some flashes of light coming from your window, wanted to know if you're okay. He laughed and said come on up for a second. Upstairs Ethyl was sitting on a chair below some extremely bright floodlamps, huge painted face topped with an enormous wig shaped like a bundle of laundry. I said hello and gave Peter the book and left. At the door I turned to him and said, It's gonna be a great decade. Ethyl shouted: I HEARD THAT!!!

⋆David moved into Peter's loft after Peter died and lived there until the end of his own life.

[No date]

I stopped in at this restaurant down on 2nd Avenue, sat at the counter for a moment and ordered a cup of coffee, feeling kind of warm and happy, the remnants of some dream from that morning still in my head. I'd pushed through something in the dream, the character of myself in the dream had arrived at a realization of how wonderful living was. All this utter seriousness having dropped away from me, I was rushing around in the dream, in some suburban landscape, through alleyways, up around garages and sides of buildings stopping people I hardly knew and telling them how happy I was. At some point I found myself with a Super-8 movie camera in my hand and it was almost nighttime and there were these two kids. I was standing at the edge of a backyard, two kids in cowboy outfits, realistic Stetsons, and pearl-buttoned shirts, setting a huge bonfire on the grass. They rushed back and forth collecting twigs and branches and even a chair, and at one point rushed back to toss them on the flames. I was seeing all this through the viewfinder of the movie camera and recording it. The colors of the flames and the light reflecting against the white wall of the garage were burning first bright oranges and reds, then these phosphorescent blues. One kid turns towards me and runs across the dark grass, becoming a silhouette against the roaring fire, rushing towards me and pulling out this gun, lifting it to the air and the light of the fire or some unseen streetlamp catching it, making it extremely bright, reflective. The look on the kid's face, movements of his body, like something strangely older than himself, he looked like some thug, some character in a small western town, sitting on a side street staircase, a bottle of wine inside a paper bag, drunk but extremely sharp in attention, beautiful looking but inclined towards violence or tension, a look in his clear eyes that seems foreign and can't be ignored. The film runs out in the camera at this point and I woke up, at first slightly confused at being in the waking world with hot sunlight flashing through the room each time the morning breeze tossed the curtains up slowly towards the ceiling, then feeling the energy of that happiness experienced in the dream.

So while waiting for the coffee to make its way to the counter, I stepped over to the phone and rang up Jesse. Zoe answered the phone sounding a little wired on something: Ohhh . . . Hi, David, I'm over at Jesse's

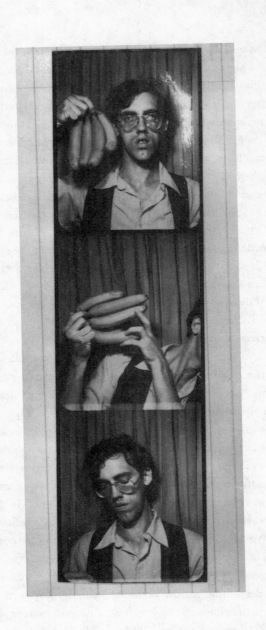

house, I've taken four quaaludes and I'm taking nude photographs of Jesse. Are you coming over? I'll take photographs of you, too . . .

I laughed and said I wasn't sure, I was just sitting down to coffee and she said, Well, I'm hideously depressed and so is Jesse and we're drowning in each other's sorrows, but we're doing art, I'm taking pictures, why don't you have your coffee and then come over? I said okay and hung up and returned to the counter and sat down. Ten minutes later I headed out and down towards the Bowery, over to 1st Avenue and then left onto Houston Street. Traffic was moving around and against the lights of the Avenues. I could see characters drinking on benches on the traffic islands.

Walking down Ludlow Street there were some little kids running around a radio playing thumping rap music, something beautiful in the characters hanging out, like summer really had arrived, street sounds like cars bucking over potholes and radio music and soft chatter of men and women on stoops. I went up to Jesse's place; Jesse left to go into the hall-way to take a piss, he was wearing this thin bathrobe. Zoe was inside staggering around, half-turning and moving into my arms hugging me: Do you want a quaalude? No thanks. Do you want something to drink? Nah, I'm okay. Jesse came back in and took off his robe and sat on the bed with his back to the wall; the building was old so the walls were plastered and painted white with some stucco effect, the kind of stucco that you could cut your wrist on if you brushed against the wall carelessly. The television was set on one edge of the bed giving off this luminescent blue light on the sheets, on the smooth surface of Jesse's chest and belly and legs. Zoe was weaving and staggering, trying to clip a lamp onto a water pipe next to the bed that ran from ceiling to floor. She almost fell backwards a couple of times and Jesse finally helped her. She picked up this long string of tin-seled garland and strung it around the bare plaster legs of a mannequin, the bottom half of this store dummy Jesse had probably found somewhere on Orchard Street. She stepped back and Jesse propped the legs by his side and pulled the garland around his shoulders: it was unsettling, the beauty of his eyes in the light of the television and the reflection of the blue light against the garland, his chest smooth and luminous in the shadows. Zoe pulled out her camera and started taking photos saying: Oh yeah . . . fuck . . . hold it . . . hold it . . . oh. Jesse would move around changing his posture, moving his legs around out of range, watching, taking pictures mentally. At some point Zoe slipped off the bed where she'd been moving around, stumbled a couple of times, and we all laughed. She finished one roll of film and sat down to reload. Jesse got up and lifted up the television in the darkness of the room and crossed the floor with it to place it down against another corner of the room. Just this luminous part of his belly and chest, arms silhouetted, the air around him, the slight haze of smoke from my cigarette turning a seedy blue, a grainy blue . . .

I finally asked Zoe for a quaalude and took it and the phone rang. It was Brian calling, he said he was going to come over in a few minutes. While we waited for him Jesse pulled out his tape recorder and picked up a sleazy pulp novel from a nearby chair, something called *Hot Hips* or *Love Is My Business,* or some such. He began reading a passage from it: And he took her breast suddenly into his hot mouth and sucked on it till the nipple seemed like it would pop off . . . Zoe and I started making these moaning sexual sounds in the background as he read, groaning enthusiastically and sucking in our breath and giving out little yips and cries of passion. The drug started hitting me and after the recorder was put down I went into the kitchen for a glass of water or tea or something. Zoe passed by and went into the other room, lay down in the darkness and called for me to come in. She told me to lay down beside her, and I did.

There was an airlessness in the room, something tight about the space, the distance between walls, the floor was one of those on which you could place a marble and it would begin rolling until it smacked against the wall, something about the time of day, the darkness making the space even smaller, the heat from the spring streets coming in through the window behind the curtains. When Zoe walked on the bed she did so with jouncing steps, she turned in midstride after I had walked in and said, Oh, I'm so fucked up, depressed but I took a bunch of quaaludes, and me and Jesse are taking pictures.

What are you depressed about? I asked, placing my arm around her shoulder. Oh, everything is fucked up. I wanna save some money, a bunch of money and leave the city, go to Australia or something.

So why don't you just save the money? Are you saving any?

Yeah, she said, Except sometimes I'm bad . . . She pulled up the white sleeve of her shirt revealing a large extended bluish bruise that started just below the crook of her elbow and ran up her arm five inches. She tapped the bruise several times like one does when they're fixing to shoot up. I've actually been pretty good, I've cut down to half the amount of coke I was shooting before.

Look, I said, hugging her, I don't understand why you people feel depressed. I've been walking around all day feeling extremely happy. I mean there's so much great stuff in living, there's so much to see and do and feel great about (I was beginning to disbelieve myself, explaining it, verbalizing it wasn't the same as feeling it, it was more personal). But I've been having these dreams, man, really, these dreams where I'm a little blond boy and I'm in this school, and they want to make me a Nazi. They make me wear these little black leather shorts and they're chasing me around like they're real strict . . .

Later Jesse came back into the apartment: Zoe's flipping?

When she lay down in the other room, I leaned in and said, Are you okay?

She said, Yeah, yeah, I'm fine. What about you?

Fine, just fine, I answered.

Come on in here, she said. Lay down for a minute. I went inside. There were clothes strewn about the floor, slightly illuminated from the bare bulb of the kitchen. I first sat down on the edge of the bed. I knew there was something faintly sexual taking place. I felt like I could see myself. I lay down, stretched out beside her, and one arm was beneath me, I think I took off my glasses, looked at her closely and said, What's up? knowing somehow what was happening.

Give me a kiss, she said. I kissed her, and she leaned back a little. Jesse was replaying the tape in the other room, we could hear fragments of sentences, some loose erotic words that sounded false, the moans and breathing Zoe and I had made behind them. Tell me about yourself, she said.

I started a short laugh. Well, uh . . .

No, I mean not where you were born and all that. Tell me what you feel about people, I mean sometimes it seems like you don't really like some of us . . . you . . .

No, it's not that, it's just that I'm sometimes distant.

Yeah, I know. Why?

Well, sometimes . . . well . . . because I have a lot of things that I love and that I respond to, and that I think about and care about and most of the people I meet . . . most of the people I know, even though I like them and have good times with them, they don't think about the same things or else they don't talk about them, share the same concerns about them that I do. Most of the people I run into are very superficial, and because I have this whole area of myself I can't share or talk about or find someone who feels the same as I do, because of that and because I don't want to lose that part of myself, I just get distant. I feel so different from most people I know . . .

She leaned forward and we kissed again. I let my tongue move across her lips, they were very small and beautiful. I felt amazed at how small she was and I started feeling an erection. I felt slightly unsettled, I hadn't done anything like this in years and years, part of me was confused at touching her, at the sense of her body which wasn't anything like bodies I was used to lying against, it was like this whole other series of movements that I wasn't quite sure of how to respond to. I was very gentle.

After a while I stopped and leaned up on one elbow and stared at her. I know, she said, You only like boys . . .

No, that's not it. Well, yeah, no, like I've been going with guys for so long, I don't know what this means. I mean I'm enjoying this, I'm feeling this, but I'm trying to understand it, what it means . . . ah maybe I'm just thinking too much, I don't know.

Well, I'm not into conversion. I just don't know about you. I mean, when I first saw you at Danceteria, I said to myself, Uh ah, don't touch that boy. I mean, I figured you were into guys but I wasn't really sure if that was all . . .

Well, I said, I . . . if I do respond to you, I mean if I could, I just don't understand what that would mean to us.

Well, she laughed, it doesn't mean that you're my boyfriend or that you'll be my boyfriend. We started kissing again and at times when I didn't think about it I would get an erection and then when I thought of her, how I knew her in context of the past year, how I'd always thought she was the most beautiful woman I'd ever seen, how I saw myself seeing myself lying on a cot with her, with my arms around her, seeing my body in that position, the cool white of her skin in the darkness, the effect of the drugs, I'd start mentally backing off, slight confusion, the sound of the tape in the other room and the hello from the other room, the laughter listening to the tape . . .

I leaned back suddenly and said, Maybe we should go out there and join them . . . She pushed me away suddenly and said, Ah get out of here. You're just another scared boy. She looked a little angry, continued pushing me away from her, but I wouldn't let go.

Leave me alone, go on . . . don't touch me, she said.

Wait a second, I'm just a little nervous. I still don't know what this means. I mean, you know I'm pretty naïve when it comes to girls.

She laughed slightly. You know that's not true. She continued pushing at me, and I started unbuttoning her blouse. Stop it, she said. You don't have to do anything.

I know, I said. I just won't think anymore. I'll stop thinking, and I passed my tongue over the surface of her breast. And we made a quiet and silent love, and afterwards Jesse came into the room with his robe open and with a slight hard-on and leaned over the two of us, laying across us on the bed saying this almost inaudible Ohh . . .

Early in the morning in a coffee shop on 2nd Avenue and 11th Street, this dive coffeehouse where gunshots occasionally ring out and pimp types are murdered, drug stuff, petty gangsters, I'm sitting there in the fluorescent light watching the dawn come up, this strong sunlight over in the trees of the church on the uppermost parts of buildings yet the asphalt street below, the cool stone walls of the cemetery of St. Mark's Church, everything cool blue like early dawn, a clarity that's unreal, and these drag queens, three of them lifting their skirts up to the traffic, wind billowing up beneath the skirts, their brown slender arms waving, pulling the skirts almost over their heads, shaking their pantied asses at passing cars, laughing loudly, small shrieks: Oh baby! Lips painted and stretched against white teeth, one guy in the coffee shop, a fat white guy with faded blue tattoos on his huge sagging arms: Lookit them faggots. They get desperate after the sun comes up. One queen comes in assuming this overly feminine posture at the counter, leans towards the fat man: Order me a cup of tea, baby. I'll be right back. Pats the place on the counter where she wants her tea and walks out, cuts up in the street laughing, fat man says to the Greek behind the counter: A cup of tea, she'll be right back in . . . cup of tea, y'hear me? And she comes back in and sips at the tea after pouring a pound of sugar in and a dash of milk and her friend comes in and takes a few sips patting their lips with napkins, first one points to this cute counterman and says, What's he, Puerto Rican? Says something in Spanish. Naw, says the fat man, Egyptian. Oh, says the drag queen. Oh, I've always wanted to take a trip up the Nile.

I turn to a guy next to me: These characters are great. Yeah, says the guy, except when they get rowdy. Other morning one pissed off a guy and the guy backed his car up and rammed forward, knocking her ten feet into the air. Haven't seen her around since then . . .

David made very few diary entries between 1980 and 1987. During that time, his career as an artist took off, and he had several solo exhibitions in New York and Europe. As well as making paintings, photographs, and films, he continued to write.

1984

January 31, 1984

In this sleep I was talking to this nice guy about thirty-eight years old with an Arizona Texan weathered face. He was all seriousness and half smiles and I turned away from him at some point realizing I had just walked on the moon and could remember parts of it, the close space of the vacuumed helmet, the sense of this time in my life realizing fully this was *me* in this suit of skin containing bones muscles blood brains, these are my hands swinging slow and smooth in some gait like a polar bear swinging these legs slow slow slow over gray grainy dusty lunar rocks and the gray-blue light in front of me beneath me stretching into distance I was giddy with my breathing and my chance to walk these scratchy dead plains with all that life, the way one keeps a favorite pebble after a long walk in a foreign countryside because of all the life one injects into it all the pleasures sensations of the body adrift in an environment away from all that drives one crazy . . .

He's just finished interviewing me and a decision's been made that I and six others will at different times be returned to the moon for a longer number of days. I am excited beyond belief. I feel extremely happy like my whole former life has suddenly dropped off like a glove—not the people I know and care about, just the feelings I carry about myself. I am stopping friends and acquaintances and telling them the news. I run into Steve my brother and tell him and he is disbelieving and then shocked but it changes his sense of me I guess. I am some homosexual living in New York and he's had some sense of connection with me 'cause of birth from the same body and suddenly here I am going to go to outer space in a vehicle I don't have to pay for.

Later there is an odd moment on the top of a staircase in a building when I've just gotten a tattoo on my chest of burning buildings and strange dinosaur monsters thrashing around one looking vaguely like an eagle but a very expressionistic tattoo and I look down holding my arms around my belly and seeing it upside down then in a mirror and it looks okay. I've let the tattoo guy go to town with his own vision, it ain't exactly mine. In that odd moment I suddenly realize: This is permanent and there forever and always and never to be removed unless I can dig up the hundreds of dollars to remove it by laser and with the size and scope of this one that would cost prolly about 40,000 bucks. And in that moment of thinking Why the fuck did I get this thing put on my chest—I became aware of the two levels of sight I have always moved on in my life: the primary one neglects all thought of future or past and I move in an excited state through events and choices of movements. The secondary sight usually involves regret, seeing the primary sight as impulsive, stupid and with reverberations of trouble, never realizing implications or consequences until the act is done. Somewhere in here comes the fear of rejection and punishment. Will they allow me to the moon if they realize who I am completely?

February 1984

I was meant to be a thief—growing up I traveled some of those roads for a ways and then backtracked and relearned my possibilities of functioning in a less horrendous way among my peers and neighbors. But the process of self-education lost contact with societal education and now years later I realize I am stranded as if on a barely drifting boat caught in the fog of a body of water in between two lands whose distance I do not know. Drifting so that it's too late to return to old ways and too little knowledge of communication to go on to new ways. A traveler without a country without a base, the map long ago switched for a piece of paper whose language and charts I cannot understand.

November 13, 1987
DREAM

I unlock a door of an apartment, it's a small studio with one partial wall separating the windowed room from the front door hallway. I'm inside without
locking the door, wondering if I've locked it. I hear a sound of some person
as I come in the door. I turn, it's night. I look toward a wall shielding the
front door, no one there. I feel a slight shiver of fear. A bed nearby. This
isn't my apartment. I've come through the night streets of a foreign city some-
place and someone is allowing me to stay in this room/studio. Tom R.★
lives downstairs directly below in an identical studio. Suddenly this guy comes
around the wall and pushes me backwards onto the bed. I am pushing him
with my arms but he's too strong and heavy. His silhouette is muscular, but
he's entirely covered in small spots of Kaposi's cancer. He's wearing no shirt,
he has an almost shaved head. He lowers himself onto me and opens his mouth
in some sort of grin, his teeth are rotted and wet, saliva spilling from behind
them. He leans close to my face to kiss me, first saying, You would have
thought I was sexy and cute if you had seen me before I got ill. I'm upset but
I give him a quick kiss so he won't think I'm rejecting him completely because he has AIDS. I feel sorry for him just briefly, but I push him off me
and rush out the door into the hall and staircase. I get downstairs to Tom's
apartment door and push the bell/buzzer wondering if it's loud and if it'll
alert the guy upstairs as to where I am. A bell rings. I push it again and it no
longer works. I'm frightened, start banging. Tom opens the door. Oh god,
I tell him. You won't believe what just happened.

★Tom Rauffenbart, David's lover since 1986, is the executor of the David Wojnarowicz estate.

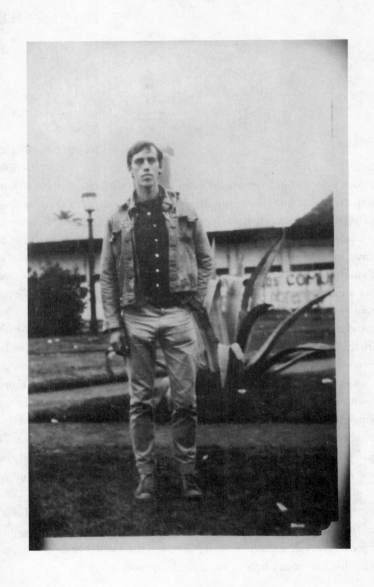

Peter Hujar was diagnosed as suffering from Pneumocystis pneumonia and AIDS on January 3, 1987. He spent the following year undergoing medical treatments. On November 26, 1987, he died of complications accompanying AIDS. Three days later, he was buried in Gate of Heaven Cemetery in Westchester County.

1987 (or thereabouts)

Peter's death. On the third night after his death it began to sprinkle rain very light. I had met Kiki Smith at a memorial at St. Mark's Church for Keith Davis who died in July. His was the first Death I'd ever witnessed. In some odd way, witnessing his death prepared me a bit for Peter's, though I wasn't as emotionally connected to him as to Peter.

I realized Peter was many things to me, or I realize it now. Peter was a teacher of sorts for me, a brother, a father. It was an emotional and spiritual connection such as I never had with my family. Maybe with my sister [Pat], as far as some real and deep connection. I remember her reading a book behind a Jersey gas station—Lee's gas station, Lee, a handsome man with grease-covered hands and arms, and a cigarette machine where I bought Dad's Lucky Strikes for 35¢ a pack. She, reading to me and to my brother Steve to calm us. We had run away from one of Dad's beatings.

My connection to Peter in this time and space we call daily living . . . I can't form words these past few days. Sometimes I think I've been drained of emotional content, from weeping or from fear. Have I been holding off full acceptance of his dying by first holding a mane camera—that sweep of his bed, his open eye, his open mouth, that beautiful hand with a hint of gauze at the wrist, the color of it like marble, the full sense of it as flesh, the still camera portrait of his amazing feet, his head, his face, his eye, his folded hands. Now maybe I'm holding his death away through impulsive ritual, not any prescribed ritual but driving north on a gray day filled with random spots of rain on a dirty windshield, all those bird nests high in the winter trees, everything rich and wet and black and brown, the serious rich black of his photographs almost wet looking, kicking around the cemetery mud among huge lifeless tractors and the ravines they made strewn with boulders and wet earth talking to Mum first walking around trying to find him. So difficult. I started to laugh nervously—maybe I can't find you—and this erratic walking, pacing back and forth from his soil, the ground to the car, cigarettes lit, camera taken back for a picture of Neal's flowers. He loved flowers, months and months of illness and the house filled always with different flowers, some so big and wild they looked not like flowers but like sentient beings, something from lunar slopes or big pick-weed fields or cow hills all wild and scrubby. All erratic movements till I stopped myself, forced myself to contain my movements, walking backward and forward at the same time, realizing in that instant how rattled I was. I was talking to him. I get so amazingly self-conscious talking to him, a thousand thoughts at once, the eye hovering in space inches from the back of my head, myself seeing myself seeing him or the surface of him, of wet tossed earth, and further seeing his spirit, his curled body rising invisible above the ground, his eyes full and seeing him behind, me looking over my shoulder, watching me, looking at the fresh ground where he lies buried. I see white light, fix my eyes to the plowed earth and see a white powerful light like burning magnesium covering the soil, his body in a semicurled position surrounded by white light floating hovering maybe three feet from the ground. I try talking to him, wondering if he knows I'm there. He sees me, I know he sees me. He's in the wind in the air all around me. He covers fields like a fine mist, he's in his home in New York City, he's behind me, it's wet and cold but I like it, like the way it numbs my fingers, makes them white and red at the knuckles. Cars at the roadside and long valleys and ridges and everything torn up, uprooted, all the wet markings of the earth and the tractors, all these graves freshly developed and those giant wet-leaved bird nests like they've been dropped by hands into the crooks of tree limbs and leafless branches. I talk to him, so conscious of being alive and talking to my impressions of him, suspending all disbelief. I know he's there and I see him, sense him, in the hole down there under that earth's surface. I sense him without the covering of the pine box, the box no longer exists in my head. It's not till later that I realize I didn't see the box just huge wide earth and grass and fields and crowfoot trees and me, my shape in the wet air and clouds like gauze like gray overlapping in fog and I tell him I'm scared and confused and I'm crying and I tell him how much I love him and how much he is to me and I tell him everything in my head, all contradictions, all fear, all love, all alone, and how I don't want him to stay around, how I wish him love and safety, feelings of warmth and beauty outside language, that I hope he will be helped and make the connections he needs so much, make the connections so that his travel will be quick and sure and that he reaches all that none of us know but instinctively some of us sense is behind that event called death— I start crying. I wish I could just touch your head, put my hands on your head . . . I'm happy for him, I tell myself at times. I feel so sure of what he's experiencing that . . . that nun that rushed into the room flinging open the door with one knock and chattering away about now you/ he accepted the church or god or something in his final days and she's chattering nervously about some text, chattering some text at me about a man she did not know and all I could feel is helplessness. I think of this guy lying on the bed with outstretched arms, I think how he's so much further there than this woman and her text, he's more there than the spoken forms, the words of spirituality. I mean just the essence of death, the whole taboo structure in this culture, the whole mystery of it, the fears and joys of it, the flight it contains, this body of my friend on the bed, this body of my brother, my dad, my emotional link, this body I don't know, this pure and cutting air, all the thoughts and sensations this death produces in bystanders is more spirituality than any words we or I or she can manufacture. The meaninglessness of words these past few days . . . I'm standing there trying to talk to him, maybe to give him something in the form of words. If energy disperses and merges with everything around us can it immediately know my thoughts? . . . So I try to speak, to tell him something maybe helpful in case he's afraid or confused or needs a tool. I want to talk about light, move towards the light, move towards warmth, but the words tip out of my mouth and immediately I know there's no meaning to them, to have meaning they have to have necessity, but they haven't that, I know, he already knows all this. I know he's beyond it already. It's maybe me that needs reassurance. I open my mouth to form words to talk, all I can do is raise my hands from my sides in helplessness and say, I need some sort of grace, and water flows from my head.

I step through the slight rain into the area before the doors of St. Mark's Church. I see candles on a table and figures moving about. I suddenly feel odd, fish out a cigarette, light it in the mist, walk to the shadows near the edge of the overhang, see people I know or don't know, silhouettes of them passing by through the bars. One waves at me as he enters the church. Finally after a second cigarette I walk into the church, someone touches me from behind, I turn and it's Kiki and the look on her face makes me start to cry again and we hold each other a long time. Later after the memorial I have this urge to go back to Peter's. It's late in the evening, Kiki and I have coffee nearby in a restaurant of stained glass, and it's the third day, the end of the third day, the papers Lynn Davis gave me say it's the time for the spirit to leave the body. Peter wanted not to be embalmed, but to be wrapped in cloth and put into a white or plain pine box and buried within twenty-four hours after a Catholic mass. He wanted to have time and no disturbance so his spirit could leave his body uninterfered with, the Tibetan papers said, three days of his spirit wandering, trying to communicate with people, the papers said not to do anything that would disturb the spirit, don't rush for his money or property. I made a simple altar or shrine on one of the large photograph tables near the side wall with an enormous beeswax candle, honeycomb we found in a drawer cabinet wrapped round and round.

I asked Kiki to come back with me and dance. I wanted to show Peter's spirit some joy, some celebration. Kiki said it was still sprinkling a bit. We turned on a few lights in his place; each time I come a little less of him is there. I spread his photos on the bed—all his childhood history, from a tiny one pressed into a stamped brass frame, almost indistinct, of him at seven or nine years old, I can't tell, and one of him at fifteen. I think he's in this rowboat set on the surface of a lake with beautiful summer leaves overhanging from the top of the photo and he is gesturing with his left hand whether to cover his laugh or to wave away the person holding the camera and now looking at the photograph I see it's a virtual cascade of leaves, pine or oak leaves, all of them tumbling around his shoulders, his other hand on the oar, and it's a canoe he sits in, naked but for his camper shorts and a laugh and the structure of his interior body pressing through. I first looked at this photo days ago, the day after he died, and thought, How could his mother not love this boy? As I spread some of his history across the surface of the bed, with the candle in the shrine burning, I put on the record Lynn found that we tried to use for his funeral mass—Tomaso Albinoni Adagio, G minor, and Kiki and I tried to waltz. I felt so extremely fraught, self-conscious, trying to follow her simple foot movements, one large step sideways, two small movements of feet, one large again, turn, swing large. Finally we shut all the lights off, started the record again, tried again, at times my whole body disappointingly shut down, all emotions shut down. I wanted to dance so freely but all this stuff of years circling over my shoulder . . . Finally Kiki let go of my hands and started whirling in the space, I did the same, dizzy from not eating all day, whirling and jumping and driving through the darkness, the window curtains open with the rain roaring through the street in huge sheets and veils across the downstairs theater lights, her body whirling through the room, her bare feet, my bare feet, never any sense of collision but sometimes dizziness exploring the place with music circling loud through the room, streetlamps burning and the rain and the rain and the rain and for a moment everything went loose in my head and I was beaming some kind of joy and I was happy for him happy that he could be seeing this naïve body starting to loosen this man and woman whirling in an invisible flutter of cloth and feet.

This guy was one of the first people I ever truly trusted, this sense of him as father and brother, my real dad being some heavy alcoholic who was a sailor and hated living whereas I fear living at times. Fear and hate, hate and fear— I don't know what the difference is other than aggression.

Started seeing this woman today, started crying when I reached the point of trying to explain how I felt about Peter, what he meant to me. I told her I didn't want to cry and she asked me why, tears running down my cheeks. Because I feel fake seconds into crying. What does this mean? So, yes, this guy was like a father, but was it really that, because I also saw him as sexual, handsome, beautiful mind, beautiful body, his was similar to mine, even with twenty years' difference. He could finish my sentences, I say to people, and he could, even though I realize through talking to people that he was such a different person to different people. Some people talk to me about their relationships to me and I feel like I'm listening to a description of a stranger. Who we are and who we are to others—it's so clear how it varies. All these people carrying small parts of this one man and with some people the parts are similar, with others it's almost alien to me.

Today I drove from the appointment onto the West Side Highway through the tunnel to Brooklyn. I wanted to film the beluga whales. These whales are so beautiful. Pale, almost gray-white bodies, streaming through the sun, luminous waters of a giant tank viewed from the side in a darkened building. Peter, Charles, and I went there months ago in his exhaustion and watched them for some time. All the mysteries of the earth and stars are contained in their form and their imagined intellect. I had read a news-paper description with a photo eight months ago that made me weep. A painted newsprint photo, black and white, of a bald thirteen-year-old girl who was in a body of water surrounded by porpoises. Some organization that grants last wishes to dying children was told she wanted to swim with dolphins before she died of cancer. The lovely face she contained in the photo and the idea of animals that embodied such grace and intellect and the gentleness of it all seemed so perfect to me. I think of Peter. I think of these whales. I think of sad innocence in the face of death and the turning of this planet.

The glass case was emptied of water when I reached the aquarium, four whales were swimming in a recessed shallow pool. Some old woman told me they would fill it on the weekend. I felt disappointed and left right away. The obsession with this film and the order of things—I get confused in these moments about why things don't work when I want them to. What I want to do is so clear to me—to reflect the beauty of the world. I tend to believe in links with the workings of the world—maybe something spiri-tual—and when things stop momentarily, when I can't complete an action, I am confused. My emotions won't allow a detour or a wait. It's beliefs like this that kept me alive all these years. And it is in this season that for the first time these beliefs are falling apart. It started with Peter becoming ill.

[No date]
[Notes for exhibition]

The Futurists thought that the machine was God. Take a walk along any river in any country and one can see that the machine is almost defunct. God is rusting away leaving a fragile shell. Factories are like the shell of an insect that has metamorphosed into an entirely different creature and flown away. But the eggs left behind in the Second World War have yet to hatch, and they have an unseen effect on all that follows.

[My] paintings sometimes deal with aspects of human technology and their mirrored counterparts in nature. Some combine self-created myth with historical mythic symbols. Printed matter from daily life is used as collage, sometimes in the shape of creatures, and sometimes buried in layers of paint to suggest memory or things considered while viewing associations of information. Food posters which have an encoded meaning of consumption are used as backdrops for information dealing with consumption on a psychic or moral level.

The photographs are arranged into a series of six groups: Religion, Control, Sex, Language, Time + Money, and Violence.

[No date]

THE THING THAT'S IMPORTANT ABOUT MEMORIALS IS THEY BRING A PRIVATE GRIEF OUT OF THE SELF AND MAKE IT A LITTLE MORE PUBLIC WHICH ALLOWS FOR COMMUNI-CATIVE TRANSITION, PEELS AWAY ISOLATION, BUT THE ME-MORIAL IS IN ITSELF STILL AN ACCEPTANCE OF IMMOBILITY,

INACTIVITY. TOO MANY TIMES I'VE SEEN THE COMMUNITY
BRUSH OFF ITS MEMORIAL CLOTHES, ITS GRIEVING CLOTHES,
AND GATHER IN THE CONFINES OF AT LEAST FOUR WALLS
AND UTTER WORDS OR SONGS OF BEAUTY TO ACKNOWL-
EDGE THE PASSING OF ONE OF ITS CHILDREN/PARENTS/
LOVERS BUT AFTER THE MEMORIAL THEY RETURN HOME
AND WAIT FOR THE NEXT PASSING, THE NEXT DEATH. IT'S
IMPORTANT TO MARK THAT TIME OR MOMENT OF DEATH.
IT'S HEALTHY TO MAKE THE PRIVATE PUBLIC, BUT THE
WALLS OF THE ROOM OR CHAPEL ARE THIN AND UNNECES-
SARY. ONE SIMPLE STEP CAN BRING IT OUT INTO A MORE
PUBLIC SPACE. DON'T GIVE ME A MEMORIAL IF I DIE. GIVE
ME A DEMONSTRATION.

In New York on the way to the airport, the cabdriver, a tall aged man
who looked somewhat Indian, said he was from Trinidad, lived in New
York for twenty years: I like driving, always loved it. You work for no
boss, you're your own boss. Sometimes you wait all day sitting around
for a job but you make your own hours and I'm out on the streets when
I like, out driving. My grandfather was brought to Trinidad when he was
ten years old. Trinidad was British-owned, but we got our independence.
In Trinidad there are Chinese and white men and they control most of
the businesses: restaurants, stores, airlines, agencies. You know, things like
that. They have the money. You have the blacks and Indians, Indians from
India. You see, my grandfather in the last century, he was a boy in India
and the British men would come through India and they would give the
boys what you call candies, we called them sweeties. So the British men
would give a boy seven to twelve years old some sweeties and you know
the drug in the hospital that makes you sleep for the operation? Well they
would put that in the sweeties and my grandfather met a British man in
the Nad and the British man gave him some sweeties and he ate it and
does not remember anything after that. He wakes up on a ship heading
for Trinidad. For a while he is very scared and the British men, they give

him something to eat and some clothes and they bring him to Trinidad to plant and cultivate and farm. In India my grandfather was the son of a farmer. The British would learn this about each child and then give them the sweeties and take them away to Trinidad for what knowledge they had in their heads. This happened to many children, and eventually when my grandfather grew up they gave him a little land, a little money, and he continued to live there and he married a black woman from there and they had children. My grandfather died some years ago. When I was twenty-seven I came to New York and I have lived here ever since.

David's work was included in I Bienal de Pintura, *in Spain, 1989.*

[No date]

Feeling better today. Finally got the cycle of sleep together. Had lunch with the gallery owner, her husband/boyfriend, and her son, a sweet kid who goes to school in England. I go through a variety of emotions. She asked me if my childhood was true, what she'd read of it. She said Luis said there was some exaggeration. I was angry that he said that. He doesn't know. But I told her I no longer talk about my childhood, that I once did because I thought it was important, that as a kid I would have busted had I read an interview with an artist or writer who had experiences similar to mine, that it would have let me feel change was possible.

[No date]
Paris

Pat's having her baby. I was sleeping in the guest room and late at night I woke with the sound of a door clacking against walls and saw a sliver of light around the frame. I thought maybe she had to pee, the weight of the baby against her bladder, whatever, but sounds later woke me, doors again, and I thought how odd, Denis is usually quiet when he prepares for work. And I fell asleep again.

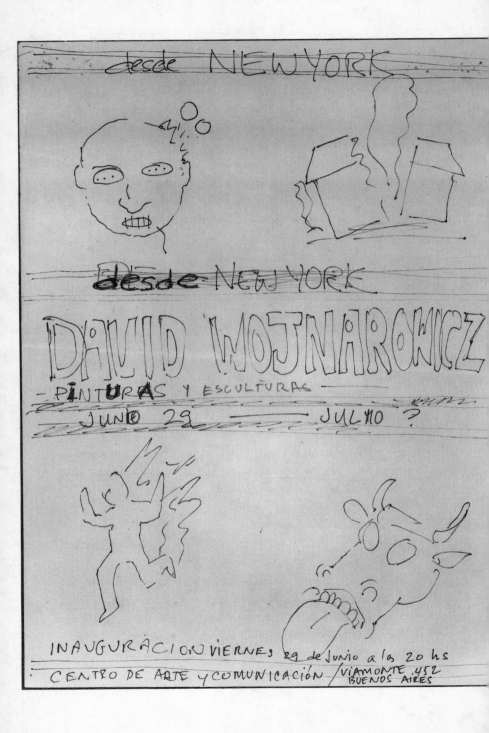

Woke up at 6:30 A.M. Denis's alarm was sounding for him to go to work. I lay there waiting for him to shut it off. Lying there with my glasses on, I was too tired to get up and say something to him. Finally I got up and walked into the hall, their bedroom door was open and the bed was in disarray. Calling out to them—no answer. It finally dawned on me that they had left and gone to the hospital to have their baby. I suddenly burst into tears. Then stopped just as suddenly as I started.

Called the clinic and asked in broken French about Denis Bernier and eventually he came on the line and told me it would be in the afternoon and he would call me when it happened and not to call back. That upset me. I felt unwanted. As if I had no right to call. No right to be there. I hung up and sat in a stunned sensation. Angry. Then breathed deep. Said out loud: I am alone. They have a separate life. I am not in that life. I feel unwanted. I want to feel wanted and loved. I feel as if I am a problem. I think Denis is stupid—a right-wing asshole with his John Wayne movies saying the movies of Israelis breaking the arms of Arab youths are just propaganda filmed in a special way to make it look like they are breaking arms. But it's really a matter of two views that are different. I won't change mine, he won't change his. We'll probably never talk about it at all. We'll never be close as in loving each other as brothers-in-law. I know that's not possible in any case. So what. I finally decide that if I want to go to the clinic I will. With or without his consent. He is not my parent. I love Pat and will move on those feelings. I feel a little tense but that's my problem. Everything is okay.

I can't go without knowing if I'm wanted there or not. All day long this tension of wondering and waiting—. I sometimes think maybe it's because I'm queer. Maybe they are afraid of what I carry, if I have AIDS or not. This fear returns often. Maybe they won't allow me to see the baby until some time. I can't imagine what it's all about. I ask myself if it's my imagination or feelings about rejection, if it's all in my head, because then it could be something that has grown out of nothing—the way I sometimes imagine the worst rejections and project them onto others who I place in power positions. It's terrible. I imagine conversations with Denis, like him telling me I can't go to the clinic. I see myself taking my bags and leaving in anger. I am unhappy with my thoughts. Angry. I want to cry and turn to someone bigger than me—emotionally or physically bigger. Am I a child again in this state?

Denis called at six o'clock. The baby was born at four. I went to the clinic. Pat was still in the delivery room, baby on a platform against the wall. I got very emotional. Tried to extend something beyond words to all of them. Later went out and walked and walked. Took photos of them all. A lot of the baby. Sweet thing. Makes more faces a minute than I did in all of Richard's movie *Stray Dogs*. The strangest thing is imagining this large creature came from Pat's belly. It's a drift back in time, then to the present, baby lying there, Pat's belly one day before, baby superimposed on memory of her (Pat's) belly, imagining baby floating in fluid, baby wrapped in cloth on a desklike surface, Pat's face weary and tearstained. Baby looks older than I imagined: pearly gray-blue eyes, one opens at a time, then both. Pat's belly, the light from the window upstairs, the color of the baby's skin, red, then faint, then red, tiny fingers with tiny nails, little working mouth. Peter. Peter's death. The shape of the earth clouds stars and space. The darkness of the delivery room shadows around the floor and ceiling all the memories in those shadows like films.

[SONG FRAGMENTS]

> *and the birds are rollin'*
> *rollin' through the trees*
> *and the forest is folding into the dark*
> *in the cradle of your hands*
> *last night I dreamed of a wind*
> *that circled around the world*
> *that blew around the world*
> *and one bridge*
> *and a bridge that touched all the continents*
> *and a sky heavy with rain*
> *and a wave that rose and covered everything*

(Was lost in some self-absorbed melancholy walking through the forest near Pat's home in the late dusk, singing these lines and drifting in the isolation and beauty of landscape and emotions when some ratty dog rushed out from under a bush and tried to bite me. Men playing cards in the grass nearby burst out laughing. Later picked up rock to throw at dog but owner put it in his car.)

[No date]
[slip of paper]

At times I feel like there's nothing to be afraid of about dying. I mean, look at how many people have done so before me.

[No date]

So I came down with a case of shingles and it's scary. I don't even want to write about it. I don't want to think of death or virus or illness and that sense of removal that aloneness in illness with everyone as witness of your silent decline that can only be the worst part aside from making oneself accept the burden of making acceptance with the idea of departure of dying of becoming dead. Ant food, as Kiki would say, or fly food, and it's lovely the idea of feeding things after death, becoming part of life in death but that's not the problem—the ceasing to exist in physical motion or conception. One can't effect things in one's death other than momentarily. One cannot change one's socks, tuck the sheets or covers around one's own body. In death one can't be vocal or witness time and motion and physical events with breath, one can't make change. Abstract ideas of energy dispersing, some ethical ocean crawls through a funnel of stars, outlines of the body, energy in the shape of a body, a vehicle then extending losing boundaries separating expanding into everything. Into nothingness. It's just I can't paint. I can't loosen this gesture if I'm dead. I fight this weariness from drugs and take a glimpse of sunlight as a conducive shot of movement of excitement of living but these drugs make me weary and frustrated.

* * *

When someone is dying in their nineties it seems somehow acceptable. Growing up I never had a notion that one need fear death. It was an extension of age, old age. Childhood memories of old people—they were ancient-looking, wrinkled like alien species, but they had familiar names like grandma or grandpa. I would think of death in terms of time—tortoises that lived 200 to 500 years old—that was enticing. Wouldn't it be great to be a tortoise? Why do we only get seventy to ninety years in comparison? But look how slowly they move. All day long eating cactus and weird plants. They can't drive cross-country, hop freights, go to the moon, except if they're dogs or monkeys strapped into a vessel by Americans or Russians—no real regard for their lives. (Monkey that wrecked capsule control panel: Hero.) In mating practices one male tortoise will knock another on his back leaving him to lie for days in hot sun till his heartbeat stops. What about cicadas? My favorite insect, living underground for seven to thirteen years, nursing like a baby at a tit, the tiny drops of water from the roots of a tree. Two weeks, maybe, of life to fuck, lay eggs, and die. Then become meaningless in that immeasurable grunge.

As a kid I thought I'd die amidst a tumble of horse legs in the dust. Some notion of wanting to live in the 1800s West, maybe beyond laws as they subsequently were formed. Less laws years ago.

I feel like it's happening to this person called David, but not to me. It's happening to this person who looks exactly like me, is as tall as me and I can see through his eyes as if I am in his body, but it's still not me. So I go on and occasionally this person called David cries or makes plans for the possibility of death or departure or going to a doctor for checkups or dabbles in underground drugs in hopes for more time, and then eventually I get the body back and that David disappears for a while and I go about my daily business doing what I do, what I need or care to do. I sometimes feel bad for that David and can't believe he is dying.

Smack makes everything so black that it takes a long long time for things to come back to your eyes. That's what I remember about it.

Looking in the eye at the possibility of real death, I haven't gotten all religious (I got as much spirituality as a humpback toad). That's not being sarcastic just that if I believe in God it's innately and that's okay. (I mean I love the idea of invisible angels walking little kids to the river and back or steadying them as they walk along a branch 200 feet above the forest floor. I even like the idea of little plastic bug-eyed saints doing magic looking like assembly-line zombies in rows by the dozens in the botanica.)

The idea that nothing matters or that nothing means anything—that's bullshit. You take a gun (that's extreme) and shoot someone: it means something (at least to them). You touch something (that's subtle): it makes a change maybe not gigantic but it does shift things, displaces air or space or thinking. Who the fuck knows what it all means? Who cares? It's all happening anyway with or without you (that's the thing about watching someone die, you turn from the deathbed or the sidewalk and then look out the window or down the street and the world is still in motion and that's both a tragic and a beautiful part of it). And days come and go and 3,000 miles away the crust of the earth spins just as fast and everything you feel and translate into images or writings can at least make someone else in the world feel like they're not alone or not crazy 'cause they feel the same things. Experience is valuable.

The only hero I have or can think of is the monkey cosmonaut in the Russian capsule that got excited in space and broke loose from his restraints and began smashing the control board. The flight had to be aborted.

Dreamt I was telling or about to tell my sister or brother that I had ARC. Started crying violently. All this tension of telling her or him almost like I had just got the news. Dream disappeared before I did.

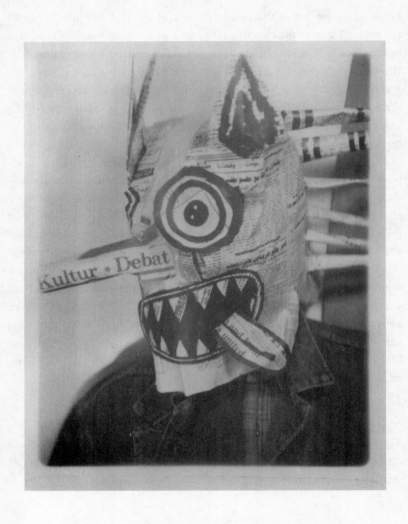

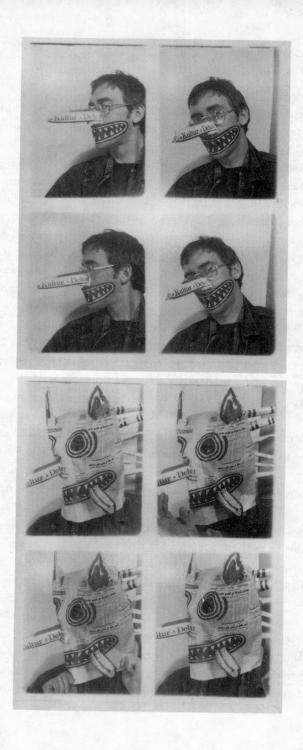

November 9, 1988

In this sleep it was some guy from ACT-UP. Never really saw him before but it made sense and he's trying to organize an action and I'm falling in love with him but thinking I've got ARC and that prevents it or prevents me from being acceptable or attractive. At some point I'm witnessing an ACT-UP meeting only it's outdoors and indoors at the same time. Some aggressive lesbian is treating this guy like his ideas are a waste of time. I finally tell her to shut up and that if she continues I'm going to have to raise my voice. I feel this is socially dangerous, that I'll be rejected if I do by the group but I go ahead anyway and in doing so I realize I hate the Right and that there is support or at least acknowledgment and she goes away, disappears into the crowd. The guy pulls me over onto a platform semiprivate on the street but somehow like a bedroom, a sense almost of privacy. We kiss and he's flirting with me touching my arms and shoulders taking small kisses. I'm very attracted to him sexually but it's more than that I feel like he'd love me and even protect me take care of me and that makes me feel very happy but then I think of my diagnosis. Scene shifts. We're near a series of large fences being constructed. He goes over to one and with another guy (who may be a construction worker but I mistake him for an ACT-UP member) he scales the fence partway then leans back pulling the top of the fence almost to the ground. It's like he is showing me how to perform an intended action. Construction boss comes running and I tell the guy to stop. Suddenly we're in a construction shack. He's got no shirt on and he's pulling me on top of him to kiss, workers all around and boss is too and some make fun of our homosexuality and anyway we answer some of their questions about our sexuality while kissing, etc. I'm really nuts for this guy, desire so strong it's a matter of being happy the rest of my life. Scene shifts. We're getting on an escalator that's miles up into the sky with the sense we're going up over a side of a very high cliff, large cables looping through rings on the sides near where our hands rest. We go up several levels, twenty stories it feels like, and crowds of people all around, at some point the escalator breaks into different upward directions. I find myself on the opposite track going towards a tunnel. A guy is moving on another track. We're about to be separated. I get upset and try to climb up to his track with a pull-up motion, got my hands on the banister, metal cable is pulling me along but I have no strength to pull myself over. He's trying to pull me over. Wall is coming up where I'll be knocked down and fall several stories. He pulls up cable ahead of me and loops it in a way to stop escalator, a knot. I get over but escalator has stopped and I get worried knot will cause cable to snap and I think of people getting killed by its snap and escalator suddenly continues and I'm still wondering how the knot was undone and I realize the guy is disappearing above me. I see the coolness of his white T-shirt. Suddenly I've arrived at a place where everyone is waiting in line in semidarkness for an elevator or something to continue the upward ascent. It looks backed up, lines of people. I feel upset and need to find this guy also wondering when I'll tell him about my diagnosis. Suddenly the gladness I feel with contact with him turns to memory of Tom. Sadness and feelings of love for Tom. I think that I don't want to lose him. I can't envision breaking up with him. I wake up sad and exhilarated simultaneously.

David was out of contact with his mother, Dolores, for most of his adult life. He had received a letter from her, to which he responded with the following, but he probably did not send it.

February–November 1989

February 22, 1989

On my way to Dallas. Who am I? Who are you? These questions, I'm wondering if I can write this stuff without including all its references. What is this mind I carry in this body? Last day I saw myself as a moving man of nerves and love and fears and anxieties and need and contradiction. I was at the gallery and Barbara Kruger sticks her head in the door to say that the work I'd done is great. What that meant to me emotionally—. Who is she? telling me she cares for my work or that my work has an effect on her— It's in the midst of my facing my mortality, I need so much in terms of what gestures I make in my work. I put all this stuff out there in a state, a whirl of sensory examination, and what is it I want or need? I want to open a window on my soul on my body on my loves and anxieties. I want to open a window on who and what I am. I want to create a myth that I can one day become. I want to adjust myself through my work—the compelling need to see the strength outside of myself before I can become it, embrace it. And simultaneously wanting to be anonymous, wanting to be faceless. The two desires can't click can't merge can't exist together. As an artist or a writer, I can at times be faceless and thus anonymous, but I really don't want anonymity. To get feedback you can't be completely anonymous. So what can I do? I am what I do, but not really. I get angry at the pressure of strength. I get resistant to the idea that I should be clear and strong in this part of my life. I want to be raw, I want blood in my work. This is why I don't revise my writings very much. Why I stop short of the ideal construction of painting or photo or whatever . . .

PETER MADE PHOTOGRAPHS
PETER HAD SEX WITH MEN

PETER HAD SEX WITH WOMEN
PETER MADE PHOTOGRAPHS
PETER COOKED FOOD
PETER ATE HEALTHY FOOD
PETER WENT TO PERFORMANCES
PETER WENT OUT ON HALLOWEEN
PETER MOVED AMONG THE RICH
PETER MOVED AMONG THE POOR
PETER MADE PHOTOGRAPHS
PETER LISTENED TO MUSIC
PETER EXPLORED THE WAREHOUSES
PETER DREAMED
PETER WEPT
PETER FUCKED
PETER PHOTOGRAPHED
PETER MADE MOVIES
PETER HAD AIDS
PETER DIED

All this stuff life is made of

[No date]

(Driving between Albuquerque and Holbrook, Arizona) I felt something loosen what with the long barren interstate and the slow withdrawal from population. It eases the eyes to see just dirt and rocks and low scrub bushes for miles and miles and clear to the smoky blue horizon. There's just rising buttes and sandstone formations and it's Krazy Kat country and in the late part of the day the trucks come shimmering through the distance bouncing sunlight off their metallic bodies into my face and beyond. Then the sun almost set and it's getting pale yellow at the horizon and the earth is turning red deep red and purple and there's tiny little cows the size of peas black against the red landscape and dotting the hills and slopes beneath the enormous Erector Set electric stanchions that look vaguely fetishlike, like kachinas

of the industrial world. And somewhere out in all that distance I feel something slipping in the back of my head. I am a member of the industrialized
tribe, the illusory tribe that catapults this nation, this society into something
thick and hallucinogenic. What is this in these wrists that grab the driving
wheel? What blood flows through these arms and hands? What color and
sense in the blood? What do these views have in common with electric
wiring? Looking through the windshield into the horizontal distance, the
scrub-dotted plains, the gray-black slopes of sudden mounds of earth appearing on the ocher and green yellow plains, the soft buttes and mountains
in the distance—what can these feet level? what can these feet flatten? what
can these hands raise?

It's a shock in the dusk, the light dusty rose color of the sloping
hills, the pearly white spherical shapes of gas tanks glowing in the fading
light . . .

David's collaboration with Ben Neill, Itsofomo: In the Shadow of Forward
Motion, *a multimedia performance, was presented in raw version for four nights at
the Kitchen in New York City.*

Ben Neill Performance

Someone once said that the Ancients believed that light came from inside
the eyes and that you cast this light upon things, whenever you turned you
cast light from your eyes onto the world.

March 3, 1989
Albuquerque Airport

THIS IS A SONG FOR ANGELS
THESE ARE THE HANDS
THAT ARE FILLED WITH VEINS
THESE ARE THE HANDS

THAT BREAK THE CHAINS
FILLED WITH VEINS THAT
LOOK LIKE ELECTRIC WIRES
BUT THESE VEINS ARE FILLED
WITH HUMAN DESIRES
SWEET SEXY ANGELS
THIS IS A SONG FOR YOU
FLYING LIKE DUMB BUGS
OUTSIDE MY WINDOW
COUGHING IN THE BLUE EXHAUST
OF THE BUS STOP BELOW
WHAT CAN THESE FEET
OF MINE LEVEL?
WHAT CAN THESE HANDS OF
MINE RAISE?

David and Tom Rauffenbart also traveled to Mexico many times, on this occasion with their friend Anita Vitale.

April 24, 1989
Playa del Carmen, Mexico

Dream. I was in Times Square, the neighborhood of my childhood hustling days, only now I'm older, my present age. It was nighttime, like a Saturday night, streets crowded with strangers off in different directions, moving quickly through the streets along the sidewalks, tourists in awe of the neon and the enormity of advertisements, of characters, a definite sense of people moving with purpose or destination intent in their heads, guarded people, sullen people. At times its filmlike vision picks up movements of bodies, legs, pedestrians from the chest down, sometimes the presence of people in transit, in movement down the streets. I'm on the sidewalk on Broadway maybe a couple blocks above 42nd Street and I see a cardboard carton on a doorway step and two little birds nestlings, one smaller, less formed than the other, hopping around in tiny bird panic. I stop and pick them up and put them in the cardboard box and the littlest one's mouth opens like a baby bird does for food. It looks hungry but I think of its thirst sitting on a street heavy with soot and grime, sidewalk dirt is magnified.

Maybe it is the dark light of dawn just as the sun is rising in the east but buried behind buildings, maybe it's midnight, the light qualities fluctuate, the little bird has the beginnings of feathers, the larger one has short new feathers. I had walked away from the box and was sad, didn't think I could take responsibility to take care of them because I was consumed in the dream feeling or wondering what my purpose was being here in these streets at this moment. I had no sense of having a home to go to, no sense of how I arrived. It was like I'd been dropped into this landscape from above, like the entire landscape and neighborhood had the sense of a miniature train-set village, yet all the particular details were breathtakingly real. I crossed Broadway and 7th Avenue in the midst of heavy traffic, dodging vehicles, drivers with feet on gas pedals, heavy traffic mayhem like rush hour. I remember fragments of other people in the middle of the avenues dodging the cars as well, I got to the other side, kept thinking of the baby birds, felt I had to go back, dodged the traffic again barely missed by cars, arrived at the carton on the doorstep, saw a bird nest, thought if I would get one of my bird nests I would put it in the carton for the two birds to sit on so they would feel protected and warm. It was cold as hell, dark sky, rain, cold feeling to the light, to the sidewalks, to the air of this sleep, a masking tape cardboard cylinder in my hands or on the sidewalk. I was thinking about a bird nest and this cylinder flipped into the box, the birds climbed immediately inside of it, a little piece of cardboard or tin suddenly on top of the cylinder sealing off the thing with birds inside. I left it like that so they wouldn't get out of the carton and be killed or lost. Crossed traffic thinking I have to get an eyedropper from a drugstore to feed them water, wondered if eyedroppers were still legal in NYC, thought of bread soaked in water to feed them, found myself at 42nd and 7th Avenue facing west, rows of movie houses and the dark light of my childhood and the streets were filled with people moving in different directions. Intensity from all the movements around me but I'm surrounded by anonymity and a sense as if the streets of the entire city were empty, emptied of people, houses, automobiles, movements, and sounds. I'm magnified and I'm seeing the movie view of myself from behind. I'm seeing my upper body, the back of my head almost silhouetted against the intensity of dusk, light blowing from the west across 42nd Street, and I begin to scream. I see the grillwork of the movie marquees and the lettering of the current shows. I see the glimmering of the asphalt between 8th Avenue and 7th Avenue in the bleached out blind light as if the street were wet after a brief spitting rain and all that light is reflecting off it turning it lakelike in pools of light and I am screaming. I am screaming so loud and so deep I am inside my body and I feel the scream and it is as if I have a ten-year-old's body and that body is as full of life, full of flesh and muscle and veins and blood and energy and it all produces and propels this scream, this scream that comes from twenty to thirty years of silence. It is a sad great deep scream and it goes on forever. It lifts and swells up into the air and the sky, it barrels out into the dusk, into the west and my head is vibrating and the pressure of it makes me blind to everything but the blood running in rivers under my skin, and my fingers are tensed and delicate as a ten-year-old's and all my life is within them and it is here in the midst of that scream in the midst of this sensation of life in an uninfected body in all this blurry swirl of dusky street light that I wake up.

June 4, 1989

Drove from Tucson to Gila Bend a couple hours before dusk and stopped at the crest of some mountain watching the light fade over the curve of the earth with silhouettes of goofy cactus and desert scrub and occasional cars or trucks slicing through the silence and one flippy bat tiny one wobbling through the wind under a roadside lamp getting knocked around trying to catch insects gathering from the shadows and a bunch of honeybees trying to drink from the steel rim of the flooded water fountain some of them stupid and drowning and a sixteen-wheel rig pulled in just as it got dark and a young guy with no shirt covered in sweat and dirt and wearing cowboy boots jumped out: What's up? and kicked each tire on his truck while I held my breath and then he climbed back in and drove away and I wondered what it'd be like if it were a perfect world.

November 1, 1989

Dear Dolores,

Thanks for your letter. I was glad to hear that you're getting close to re-
ceiving a teaching license. I wish you luck on that as I imagine that it represents a big change in life direction and security. It does sound intense to
be working in the city school system. The school system wasn't any great
shakes when I was a kid so I can imagine how much worse it's gotten. The
whole city is at this point a slow dying city; I doubt the next elections will
change its direction very much. I don't trust Dinkins any more than Giuliani.
Both treat drug addiction problems with the same stupid proposals: more
cops. The street I live on is one of the many drug alleys in NYC and it's
been like this for two years and cops coast by here all the time and once in
a while arrest some junkie too sick to run fast enough. Waiting time for
treatment programs is at the minimum nine months. People sleep in tents
in the local park and now I hear they want to throw people out of the subways in winter.

I've been going through a lot of personal problems for a couple years
now and am not sure how any of it can be resolved. I'm pretty tired at
times and stopped therapy for a few months but may continue sometime
soon. I've been involved in a lot of projects related to art and video. I am
dealing with health issues in both friends and in myself. I was diagnosed
with ARC recently and have been trying to find a treatment I can physically deal with—AZT was too toxic for me to handle so I'm looking into
some experimental drug trials. I have been wrestling with the psychological
aspects of this as well as some of the social problems. Sometimes I get
involved with groups fighting city and government policies towards people
with AIDS. I also have a great deal of anger I am carrying towards events
in my life, in my past as well as what I see around me now. A fair amount
of this anger comes with the territory of facing some measure of mortality. I find it hard to tell you about all this because I have been pretty isolated for the last few years; I'm rarely that social and even with the diagnosis
of having this disease [sic] I feel it necessary to be by myself most of the
time. I'm trying to resolve some of my own feelings of self-hatred that I
carried from the early days of New Jersey and from some things in New

York. It just gets so complicated in terms of what is buried and what I come across in therapy.

Mom, I have a lot of mixed feelings towards my relationship with you. I am caught between the understanding of what problems you carried from your experiences with your family and with [?] and also with dealing with three kids, and the experiences of what I carried as a kid. There is no immediate answer for any of those things; I just have so much buried inside me that is scary to touch and at the same time I am trying to reach it when I am in therapy. I don't feel very healthy mentally although given what my life has been I am doing okay. I've hesitated telling you about this diagnosis because I need privacy and distance right now. I'm not sure when I will feel ready to get together with you because it feels so loaded with things I haven't been able to resolve. I do think of you and always hope for the best for your life and whatever things you are trying to do. I appreciate your words in the letter and wish your parents were able to write the same things to you.

I have found that even with these issues of mortality that I am facing that things aren't all that different. Maybe I appreciate things more on a certain level but I still have the same problems I have always had. There is just a little more pressure. Sometimes I feel scared and then because my health has been steady for a while I pretend that things are okay in a certain way so I can continue moving.

[No date]

Dreamt I was in a club of sorts. Tom was there, a show was about to take place onstage and I'm sitting near Tom and he is acting a bit strange. I'm not sure about the situation but it feels public in the way that has always made me tense. We are in a relationship, but some emotional part of the relationship has never fully connected, maybe because of my need to be a stranger to all events so that I can witness them without complicated emotional connections. So I can lay back in my fantasies in the process of witnessing, something extremely self-conscious in the act of witnessing, as in the warehouse days, coming through a series of abandoned rooms filled with evidence of various elements—wind, rain, rust, decomposition of plaster, etc., and also the evidence of sex acts and bodily functions such as human shit and tissues balled up with the same and occasional pairs of underwear or socks or T-shirts sometimes covered in shit or lying overlooked and abstractly human in piles of plaster and lumber or pools of rainwater—and then suddenly I'd come across two or five naked men in the throes of various leanings of sexuality, a glimpse that takes all the details in then I move on, away from the source of heat and flame.

Tom is acting aggressive, saying things to me and interrupting the act onstage, and the audience is watching us and I say I'm going to leave and he grabs onto my arm and I can't get his fingers off and he gets louder and I think he's telling the particulars of our relationship. I'm getting angry and thinking that our relationship is definitely over after this scene and all my clothes are in bags my coat nearby and maybe a camera lots of belongings to have to be responsible for and I can't even get away from the table and I start pinching his fingers. He holds on tighter and I'm yanking and pulling away but can't get away. I suddenly have a knife like a vegetable paring knife. There's a guy onstage in a spotlight doing a routine or announcing the unfolding events and I press the knife to Tom's fingers clutching my arm and the knife immediately cuts into the flesh of his knuckles and I slow down and lift the knife a bit—all as if this is irretrievable or unalterable once it happens and that upsets me deeply. I feel I have nothing to bargain with nothing to threaten him with as it's all gone too far and finally he lets go and I leave to another room without most of my things and I realize I have no shirt on, my shirt is in my hands. I'm a little embarrassed to be in public without my shirt on so I go into the men's room to put it back on. A young guy is peeing in the upright urinal. I step into an unconstructed part of the room with dangling wires and two-by-fours and a dim bulb light and the dream goes away as I wake in New Orleans—twelve hours sleeping in a shitty hotel room where the shower curtain has printed on it: ALL OUR GUESTS ARE V.I.P.S.

The window is my television set and the streets are my newspapers—

David and his lover Tom Rauffenbart traveled several times to New Orleans for holidays.

Airport (waiting)

It's that late-afternoon winter light that bathes everything in the landscape giving it an apparition of warmth. I'm sitting at a second-story table behind the plate glass of some crummy piece of architecture feeling dark. Maybe it's what we call sadness, maybe it's darker than that, and all I can think about is the end of my life. In the far distance at the edge of the runway is a thin wedge of horizon made up of dark dead brush maybe trees formless other than the rusted oil refinery or the couple of odd buildings made of blond concrete and shadows. What does it all mean? What's going on in this head of mine? What's going on in this body? in these hands? that want to wander that guy's legs over there . . .

A construction crew down below in the framed-off area of the runway asphalt: I can count eight or more of them in winter drag and helmets. I feel like shit. I guess years ago I could think of what the interiors of those trailers look like, filled with drafting tables or cheap oak furniture and calendars and ringing phones and a ratty couch and some fantasy of one of them taking me inside and locking the door and removing his sweater and thermal undershirt all in one move so I could taste his sweat but that's a drift of thought that takes effort and I don't care about making that effort. What does it mean? What for and why and the red tail fins of some of the planes parked below have white crosses on their sides and I'm afraid I'm losing touch with the faces of those I love. I'm losing touch with the current of timelessness. Maybe I won't grow old with a fattening belly and some old dog toothless and tongue hanging in the house. I won't grow old and maybe I want to. Maybe nothing can save me. Maybe all my dreams as a kid and as a young guy have fallen down to their knees. Inside my head I wished for years that I could separate into ten different people to give each person I loved a part of myself forever and also have some left over to drift across landscapes and maybe even to go into death or areas that were deadly and have enough of me to survive the death of one or two of me—this was what I thought appropriate for all my desires and I never figured out how to rearrange it all and now I'm in danger of losing the only one of me that is around. I'm in danger of losing my life and what gesture can convey or stop this possibility? What gesture of hands or mind can stop my death? Nothing, and that saddens me.

A man on the balcony takes a Kodak picture of the sunset and uses a flash. What does he hope to illuminate? If I could I'd descend the stairs and run with my eyes closed across those runways to the horizon and break through the screen of dusk like a large piece of paper held vertical and enter a whole other century or life and jump into a warm ocean and swim until I disappeared . . . Once in a warehouse along the Hudson River I wrote about a man who drove a single-prop plane out over the ocean till it ran out of gas and I envied that man and this was years and years ago so I have been living on borrowed or new time. Should I count backwards like the Mayans so I never get older? Will the moon in the sky listen to my whispers as I count away?

David took his last trip to the West Coast in the summer of 1991, on the occasion of his book Close to the Knives: A Memoir of Disintegration *being published by Random House, and the Outwrite Lesbian and Gay Writers Conference, for which he was invited to speak on a panel on AIDS and literature.*

January 6, 1991

Sleep. Some sad homeless guy telling me to bring him some citrus fruit, telling me which street by which brick wall he'd be sleeping beneath cardboard. I wanted to bring him more substantial goods but he made it clear what he wanted: oranges.

A house, a building, a barnlike structure or a gutted loft or a store on street level, broken wood slats, windows, walls broken out in the interior, men, five or more young men, nude, seminude, communal, lying around. One of them is talking to me, engaging me in conversation. It's late, lights are turned on, actually it's going towards sunrise. At first the scene looked possibly dangerous but the guy is sweet and earnest. They all look poor and just in the building, crashing. Trucks outside like circus trucks. These guys workers? The one guy, built and half naked standing up clutching a silly costume of some sort wrapped around his waist like a dress made of gold gilt fabrics dyed turquoise/silver/gold/yellow like Cleopatra 1980s floor show uniforms but now treated as blankets for sleep. At times I think this is my place or vague echoes of Patrick, maybe his friends or just his energy, vague connections to energy of university students. Waiting like someone will return to dwelling and disrupt the writing process in the dream.

Guy I'm talking to and walking with finally says, I wish you would lay down and bunch up with me, meaning embrace me, snuggle, etc., and I'm delighted. I take off some clothes, turn him over and kiss his ass cheeks and see/feel a rash or dirt, hope he is not ill with a weird disease, then it looks more like grime that one gets lying naked on an unswept floor. I kiss his naked sides, his arm, his mouth. Later he talks a lot. I wish lights would

231

be shut off so I can have privacy with him because all these other guys are awake and watch from lying positions around the room.

At some point wandering around the place, floors covered in layers of refuse, objects, clothes, torn fabrics, etc., a coffee machine or water bottle or something with wires plugged in wall, waiter trying to put water in machine and water spills and spreads like a rain puddle beneath clothes, objects, water raining down onto electric outlet, a dull buzz of electricity building muffled whoomp inside wall, afraid to go near it all, afraid of electrocution or fire. Everything is quiet. Waiting.

One guy asks me if I remember my past, if anyone has ever told me of my past. I'm trying to figure out that question, it's such an odd question. Guy I was kissing says he found out his diagnosis in '88 or something like that and he's relieved he knows I have this disease. I was afraid to kiss him too extensively before telling him. Feel a bit emotional towards him and it feels clear and good. Wake up.

I was standing in the shower rubbing my body with a bar of soap and thinking about death, thinking about sex, thinking about the drama on television last night, a courtroom drama where some guy with HIV is on trial for having sex with a woman without rubbers and she has contracted the virus and he was on the court stand trying to articulate why he didn't tell her he had the virus. He said he just wanted to make love to her; the virus didn't enter into his thoughts at that moment. I thought of the the "AIDS Monster" headlines of the *New York Post* back a few years ago: some guy on Long Island with AIDS paid a few dollars periodically to suck off the dicks of teenagers. I thought of a news story in California of a Buddhist monk who was HIV-positive and was found having unprotected sex with his followers. He was asked why he did this and he replied, I don't know, or, Because this is the world, something along those lines. And I thought of a projection into some part of what these people embody in terms of states of mind. I saw myself having unprotected sex in this projection and saying, We all will die one day, days from now, years from now, and in all the vast kinetics of the moving world of what we call life, what difference is there in my life if I die tomorrow or if I die a dozen years from now? What is the difference between tomorrow and the dozen years? What does the dozen years contain in terms of difference if you measure this against the fact that we all die? If you can tell me the difference, if you can tell me what the dozen years means in terms of the structure of death as a natural component of life, tell me what that twelve years means, tell me what it contains that makes a difference not just emotionally but in the wider structure of the planet and moving forms. If you can explain what that twelve years gives or means to a person other than a continuance of groping within a blind structure, then I can understand and enact a desire to live beyond the sad gestures of human activity which is about rejecting the concept of death. I guess somewhere I feel that the twelve years makes no difference other than an emotional abstraction of the idea of death for another twelve years—a thrusting away of death which our social structure battles with, by creating distractions, endless distractions.

When I've gone to a movie house periodically to jerk off, there are at times men who approach me and begin to lick my throat or kiss my hands or jerk off next to me or try to kiss me and I sometimes allow a measure of touch and suddenly this guy's head attempts to go further and with the weight of my hand I prevent him. I feel comfortable to take responsibility to prevent him from doing anything that is dangerous to himself, but I also recognize in that moment that he has released himself from responsibility for himself. He submits to desire which negates death for him, which negates the possibility of death. The virus is invisible to the eye for both of us in that moment, but the pushing motion of my hand against his forehead even if he struggles with all his might in order to force me to let him do what he wants, my hand is like iron, I won't let him pass this line of desire. If I were to speak and tell him I have this virus in my body, he might flee or he might be angry because he kissed my neck or licked my chest, or he might not care and want to chance doing what he wants, which is to suck my dick. Sometimes a guy will get angry at me for not allowing him to do what he wishes and then go off down the aisle and immediately start blowing someone who will let him do what he wants. Some of these guys stay all day in the movie house and blow dozens of men. Everything is in motion inside the dark confines of this theater that shows blurry porno flicks on a cheap unfolded screen, and life and death is simultaneously being hatched, structures of life and death, plans of life and death are being made by physical communications and gestures. This guy doesn't trust the idea or concept of death enough to take his own precautions, or else maybe he feels it's too late to worry because of his history and the possibility that he already has the virus and that in the mechanics of sex many people don't believe it is highly possible to transmit the virus orally if they refrain from swallowing semen. I don't know what it is he thinks but I feel safe in what I allow or don't allow in terms of touch by fingers or tongue, all of it confined to the external and the areas free of seminal contact, but it also makes me wonder about the machinations of the world and the fragmentations of social order and disorder, all shifting simultaneously and creating designs and patterns that we call the world, that we call life. And I'm still wondering what that twelve years makes in terms of a difference beyond the frail human structure we call society and the world and personal activities that make up our lives. I guess I'm still trying to understand some concept of life in measurement against the universe and life/death cycles or capsules. What does that twelve years mean? to him? to me? to all whom we interact with? What does it mean outside the time we refer to as life? What does it mean to our selves? What does it mean?

1991 (through August)

I'm not so much interested in creating literature as I am in trying to convey the pressure of what I've witnessed or experienced. Writing and rewriting until one achieves a literary form, a strict form, just bleeds the life from an experience—no blood left if it isn't raw. How do we talk, how do we think, not in novellas or paragraphs but in associations, in sometimes disjointed currents . . .

I was feeling burnt out and shitty and all I had working in my head was some little place in the brain that wills the body to find another body and fuck it kiss it lick it follow the tongue and the senses where they lead. I was coming off of speed which always left me so consumed in a search for a body that would hook into some buried dream or fantasy whether violently or passionately it wouldn't really matter which, they might be interchangeable. I didn't really know what I wanted. When I'm caught in the search for it, it is like the body is a conduit, a receptor of symbols or energy or merely moving forward drifting through the urban scenery waiting for a dozen signals to intersect the right way as to surprise, open the eyes, stir the senses, find me, and unexpected hard-on.

I was walking the streets below Times Square, around the 30's between 7th & 8th Avenues. There used to be a thirty-story office building on 7th Avenue with revolving doors locked down for the evening after the last worker had left for the day, and behind the dark glass one night at two in the morning I saw a night watchman waving his big dick at me. He unlocked the door and let me in, relocked the door and led me to a back ground-floor hallway where he had a folding chair and a little desk and a shitty transistor radio playing Latin music on a low volume. It crackled and hissed tinny music that lifted and floated in the marble and polished halls.

He pulled his pants off, folded them and lay them on the desk, pulled down his fake silk boxer shorts around his ankles, sat on the metal chair and directed me to kneel before him. I did this once a week for the better part of the summer until one night he wasn't there. I could see his little lamp burning back in the shaft of the hallway but he must have quit or got fired. He never returned no matter how many times I did.

The streets at one A.M. are very very dark up in the 30's, as if all the lights are concentrated in 42nd Street. Everything else dims in the radius spreading out from that street. Everything, each surface has a glittering quality. There is so little light that touched anything directly, as signs of life, little granules of glass in the asphalt, the sidewalks, pools of wet stuff, occasional faraway streetlights, pools of black darkness where it's hard to discern grates and barricades and doorways and burglar gates and occasionally the dim light of what seems like a fifty-foot-high streetlamp illuminating a sphere of sidewalk, piles of large cardboard boxes from factories and sweatshops hidden behind the fashion/garment district facades and showrooms. Nothing but the sound of skittering newspapers, pieces of cardboard dragging down the street, garbage spread everywhere, rotten produce in the gutter, sounds of traffic on the main avenue, occasional side street cabs bumping potholes, indiscernible click of traffic lights on empty streets, vague silhouettes of mannequins behind dark windows and solder gates, poor versions of American fashions for overseas. On 8th Avenue there's rarely a living being below 40th Street—it's maybe too dangerous or the pickings too slim to draw any interest.

Suddenly darkness moves and a human is sliding along the storefronts close to the windows and doors moving bent over with intent or with loss— something in the body language or the clothing, broke, in pain, weary, hopelessness. Cars come in twos or threes burning up the Avenue with foot pushing the gas springing from a red light that's finally changed, charging uptown giving the impression there's nothing here to stop for, people rushing from one location to another and I wish at times I could read the entire history and intentions and structure of a person to know what sad destinations they have before them in that moment.

On 37th Street on the west corner of 8th Avenue, there was an illuminated window, gates half down, a donut shop, and the apparition of a man naked above the waist mopping the floor around the horseshoe counters. I stood on the opposite corner—the image was kind of beautiful, in the periphery of sight it was just six-story buildings and empty streets, everything buried in black shadows and gritty low-level light, newspapers lifting gently in the warm breeze, the skip of occasional car wheels over manhole covers, the metallic hum of circuitry in the traffic lights and the sky that weird charcoal blur gray where night is softly illuminated from the city below. And in the midst of all this desolation a bright rectangle ten feet by twenty feet fluorescent unreality and thousands of fresh donuts stacked into the racks and a sexy Puerto Rican man, his muscular body just beginning to fade from youth softening up at the edges sweeping motions of the mop from side to side, white kitchen pants and athletic shoes and he's totally unaware of being watched.

I worried that he might beat me up if he took my presence the wrong way but also figured there were no witnesses to my desire so he shouldn't feel threatened or the need to defend his honor, being the recipient of any gaze. I walked slowly back and forth along the sidewalk. At some point his head swung up. He was remopping the floor with a dryer mop but his head dropped back down and I vanished from his perception. Next I decided to be obvious.

I stood a few feet from the main window and hands in pocket, I stared. He caught on and waved me away and went back to mopping. I figured that was it but my legs wouldn't respond. I thought I better not push it but then even getting punched would ease the lust, the pressure of coming off speed, the need for connection, to be at the hands of another, to be led into some ritual or experience where flesh connects with flesh. It's funny, the chemicals that the body can manufacture. I could feel them burning through my solar plexus into my chest my heart my neck tightening my forehead and cheeks getting hot. He looked up again and seemed mildly angry, dropped his mop into the steel bucket and unhooked a mass of keys from his waist and walked towards me. I felt like I should run but stood my ground feeling weak in my arms and legs the way you do when you're about to fight a stranger or a group of teenagers are suddenly surrounding you. He swung open the door and in an impatient manner waved me inside. It was odd stepping out of relative darkness into such illumination—someone three blocks away could see every detail of our interaction. I felt naked and stupid. What do you want? He had locked the door again but left the keys dangling from the inside lock as if my answer would determine whether he moved forward or backwards.

Uh, you.

How much you pay me?

I never did this before, never even considered it. I sold my body literally thousands of times and always thought it was sad that people paid others for the use of their mouth arms legs hands assholes chest back feet. I don't know, I said. You like to get fucked? he asked. Yeah. Twenty dollars. All I had was a ten and some change. My head was pounding from blood. I'd decided. Ten dollars you suck me. You wanna get fucked it's twenty dollars. Okay, I said, reaching into my pocket. Not here, he said. Come in the back. We walked into the kitchen area, a long steel table covered in flour and confectioners' sugar, large steel pots hanging above a stove, scents from smoke or burning food. Where's the money? First the money. His belt was black with a gold buckle. I could see the outline of his underwear beneath the white cloth of his pants, the skin of his legs slightly darker.

I thought of all the truck drivers and factory workers that would be eating 69¢ breakfasts at the counters in the other room in a number of hours. Would they taste this moment of sex of energy in their donuts, in their meals? Would they sense it having taken place and say something to the waitress? How long does the smell of sex or its energy hang in the air? I handed him the ten. It was moist. He took it by the tips of his fingers and laid it gently on the steel table avoiding the flour dust. Then he started opening his belt. I kneeled down before him so that my face was just inches away and watched his magnified hands, each detail of his fingers as they unhooked the belt and slid it open. The zipper took hours to finish its ride from top to bottom. He pulled down the front of his underwear until it nestled tightly beneath his balls and his uncircumcised dick jutted out. I moved forward and turned my head to lick his balls and his hand pushed my head away. None of that, just suck it. As I took it in my mouth both his hands grabbed around the back of my head and roughly pulled me down on it. He started pumping like a piston. I unzipped my zipper and pulled out my dick. Somewhere in the back of my head I thought of my childhood and how it made sense to pay this guy. I kept trying to understand what it was I was thinking. No images formed at all, no continuous thoughts, everything fragmented, this dick in my mouth, the earlier sense of potential violence, the mouths I stuck my dick into as a ten-year-old and the rough texture of anonymous men's hands, wedding rings, old suits, hands opening wallets, a few old bills, hotel countermen and sign-in cards, registration cards with fake names and signatures, the sweet dust of sugar in the air, his hands tightening in my hair, the close-up of the white chef's trousers like hospital pants, the black pubic hair brushing my nose and his lips, the expanding qualities of his dick, the heat it was generating, his face looking down at me with a mixture of anger and the beginning sense of losing himself entering the dark pupils of his eyes. He came. I swallowed. I came and he stepped back pushing my head away and reaching for a paper towel to wipe his dick off with. He looked at the little splash of cum on the floor between my legs and looked disgusted. I felt confused. What did he think it was I got from putting my mouth around his dick?

[No date]
San Francisco

I would like to evaporate into the walls into the surfaces of things. I'll never fall in love again. He is shocked at me saying this. It doesn't shock me. It feels perfectly natural and sane. I mean I'm empty and I feel like I am dying and when you're dying it's not like you can make plans that aim like arrows into the future through the boring walls of this crammed up existence. I'm not unhappy. Only when I feel sick I feel unhappy. I feel more like my body is in neutral. On the television set they keep doing live reports from Sacramento because of the Thrill Killer who strikes on Tuesday nights. I might not be able to stop myself from laughing if the newscaster gets thrill-killed on live camera. This doesn't mean I am cruel, just that I am empty at the moment. It is not that I am cynical it's just that I am facing reality, I guess. In a movie house today on Market Street a man in the balcony sat down next to me and pulled out a fat wet dick, I couldn't see it only knew it was there when he wrapped my fingers around it. I have to admit he was repulsive. White like a body sucked dry of blood but that dick was thrilling to hold. It kept leaking all over my fist, his hand pushing the back of my head. I became iron and silently refused his dick— it wasn't that thrilling, if you know what I mean. It was just circumstances, the little kid on the movie screen dressed like a baby Satan and the vague sound of police helicopters shuttle over the theater blaring commands that lose translation in the circuits of their loudspeakers. Dying is boring—it narrows down too much. I keep dreaming of years ago when I wanted to be a hard-assed thief in a car on a road leading to any horizon and death would be a banner waving in miniature behind my eyes in my pupils seen only by the people I kissed and chances are the circumstances would be too ill-lit to be read and my body would slam into that hustler's body, I thought he was like a swimming pool I wanted to dive right into. This neighborhood in six months has gotten dark and heavy. I walked around after getting into town and it was like a blanket of violence had descended, something atmospheric and fragmented not made up of specifics just a wound drying up on that guy's face, the skinny bony queens with fake colored hair in thin windbreakers crouched next to bushes and base-ment windows on the side street waiting for customers and abuse in the fucking chill of evening. The woman maybe sixteen maybe seventy with a catalog of beatings still bloody or fading to bruises and she's not self-conscious walking into a cheap coffee shop asking to use the locked toilet and being refused. Groups of teenagers whose eyes you bypass because of their death banners waving waving waving waiting for the wind to stop blowing or the breeze to slow down. So silken death folds and twists and embraces you tighter at the throat. It's all fragmentation nothing specific and it's reading the signs the codes the walking moving evidences buried in shadows.

Hey Dave, he said. Gosh it's been a long time. How are ya? He still has his heavy metal haircut, jet black, feathered down his face and neck. He talks kinda funny though. I wonder if he's still a crack addict. How you doin'? I asked him, fishing for words. Fine since I found Jesus, and he smiled. When his lips peeled back they revealed a cage around his teeth, an obscene structure of miniature fencing and steel tubes and silver caps and deep blood bruises for gums. What happened? Oh I got hit by a car riding my bike, wired up my jaw but Jesus is in my life. I just pray, you should try it. He loves us all. The guy he was with was nodding out on the corner. God bless ya, Dave.

It's an enormous white wall about the size of a football field standing upright on its goal made of rough bleached stone. There are only two windows way at the top. One double window on single right next to it inches away. Both black with tinted glass in the slight fog. Rich people live there; they see sights the rest of us don't see. The news for them is and will continue to be good. They are very proud of their armies halfway around the world and the work they are doing. They are proud of themselves for how they have edited their view, their lives, their neighbors, us down below. They hear very little of our lives, they hear little of our hollers our screams our hunger our choking. They usually avert their eyes from below, they can look at any hour of the day into my room, my single room in this cheap hotel. They might see me naked reclining on my bed watching patriotism on every station on the dial. They have faith in god and country and concrete and steel and limited numbers of windows usually high up where no gymnastics or ladders can reach. I could close my curtains but I want them to struggle with the intrusion of their view. Nakedness is a difficult thing for anyone to ignore. We load it with symbols which have meanings our lives supply. My nakedness shows my hunger. My image can go where my voice would falter and dissipate. The rich have shades on their three windows, long black slats of designer materials. Two slats on the smaller window are parted maybe permanently. They may be at home, they may be away, it doesn't matter. I have all the time in the world. I experiment with small explosives and crude brand-name missiles temporarily made from stove matches tinfoil and now small steel cups. There are seven or eight spots on the white wall that look like attempts at spin art. They are my previous attempts. I'm getting better. I think of the smoke I will one day see pouring like death petals from those three windows. I think of the rich hanging over the balcony, the windowsills. I think of their full bellies. I think of their useless bank accounts. I think of their armies, their soldiers occupied halfway around the world. I do things in my bed that I imagine would appear rude and without taste to them if they were home and looking downwards for a change. I wave periodically.

GUY ON POLK STREET

He looked like a cigarette cowboy who had gotten into a bad accident in the last year. Like he'd been delivered a terrible blow from the rear, something so massive and total it was like he was hit with a machete the size of a refrigerator. The result pushed his skeleton so it rested just beneath the skin on the front of his body. The eyes were the only things that remained where they originally were—way back there. His body language recalled rodeos and steer herding but was more like clichés now, like old John Wayne movies. He had no great lines (words) spill from his lips like before commercial breaks. His eyes were advertisements for early death which probably no one would notice. His death would spark and sputter like a malfunction of a halogen light.

KID ON MARKET STREET

He reminded me of those wolf children they find in remote jungles or forests of India and bring snarling and spitting to one of Mother Teresa's orphanages where he will refuse to eat, walk on curled knuckles, and sleep in a dark corner on a small rug as opposed to the downy mattress, tortured by halogen lights and media crews. He will die within the year.

When did the hard rain fall as predicted twenty-odd years ago? What language can we invent to replace that term rooted as it is in historical mythologies and dead-end media, fadeaways and blackouts? The war is close to an end interrupted by commercials for painkillers and rash creams. I'm in a cold wet city that is gasping for water in the worst way in its history and yet water makes some people miserable, the ones huddled in barely recessed doors around City Hall under wet sleeping bags. It recently became illegal to be homeless in this area after the civic center and stock exchange and department stores close up at night. Forget the "hard rain"— it takes so many forms whether carpets of bombs or the choking silence of people's invisibility. We starve or watch people starve—politely we turn channels on people's lives or deaths. We step out of their reach into autos and planes and luxuries too boring to list. A man pulled out an enormous black dick and stuck it through two heavy red velvet curtains at me and I sat with my back to it. The usher for this moist disintegrating movie house discovered him and shone a flashlight in his face until he fled into the rain. The guy with the dick should have been given a medal. It was such a lousy film and I felt an emptiness as wide as the missing sun. A kid of fourteen pressed his forehead against the glass separating us as I ate a small meal that has woken me up six hours later. If I am nauseous is it permissible to lay responsibility on the world and its movement? It feels something like car sickness only larger. The kid has a wet bundle of worldly possessions and he's looking for at the very least a hungry mouth more hungry than his own so that he can bargain. Forty Iraqi troops surrendered in the desert to a marine drone, a very small pilotless plane armed only with a video camera. My body has feet, my hands feel helpless, weary or useless when confronting the future of all this. The whole world is going on at a distance or maybe it's me who is at a distance or maybe it's me who is in the distance watching it grind to a creaking halt. How do you describe emptiness without using words? Making sound disrupts that emptiness but it isn't that easy because at some point you have to stop to breathe.

Trying to remember states of mind when I was seventeen. I'd bought a bus ticket to Ohio I think or maybe it was to the furthest state line in Pennsylvania. It doesn't matter because America had already passed the loan, destroyed itself like a self-destructive or suicidal amoeba, this was when everything was reformed and rebuilt to look the same in order to ease people's fears of foreignness and to induce them to travel without having to risk making new choices. I sat way in the back of the barely empty bus, the rest of the passengers clustered like flies behind the driver. He was sexy. I could see his face for the entire ride in the large rearview mirror. I pulled out my dick and wrote poems in my head for hours. I had a hard-on for 300 miles.

It's so odd trying to write about the past based on memory: the landscape and human particulars fall to the odd logic of time and emotional impression. The landscape of memory is as affected by time and personal structure as is landscape affected by light or darkness. At night when sources of light are curtailed, shaped, bent, deflected, erased, the distances can suddenly be elongated or shortened, physicality of self or landscape expands or contracts in the dark. 8th Avenue in memory can be a location or landscape no one else has ever traveled.

[No date]

Having this virus and watching guys having sex and ignoring the invitation to join in is like walking in between raindrops.

[No date]

AIDS IS NOT ABOUT DEATH. IT IS ABOUT PEOPLE LIVING WITH AIDS. This is bullshit. I understand the concerns about media and how it has manipulated images of this virus which can affect public perceptions and funding for research and health care. But AIDS is not just asymptomatic muscle boys and kick-boxing dykes leading the public fight against this virus. Those of us dealing with manifestations of this virus need room to embrace and look at the very real possibility of Death. Having seen many friends go through horrifying illness and die, having fevers and night sweats for the last two months, feeling horrible and fragmented, I demand that we don't slip into denial about Death as an aspect of AIDS.

In the paper today I read a story about a woman in an animal park who tried to stop a fight between two 5,500 lb. elephants. She died. Phil kept saying there's something in the paper that was hysterical. I tried to find it. The first story I read was the elephant story: "She loved elephants too much."

[No date]

So I get on the plane and everyone looks like a Kennedy and some weird excessively aggressive man sits next to me across the aisle. It's an empty plane but he's thrashing around slamming overhead doors throwing his seat belt out of the way to sit down and generally looking like he's in a rage. I imagined him a hijacker. I imagined my death at his hands or his death at mine. I must be anxious. What is all this? My hands are so sensitive, my whole body is so wound up I feel again like I want to puke or scream. I wish I was rid of this body. I wish I could leap out of this skin and run away or explode or disintegrate. I can't stand the feeling of air let alone my clothes against my skin. I have these images in my head of ripping out my veins my nerves my skeleton. People are so weird, so unconscious. The waitress is giving us pretzels with too much salt, a ginger ale that tastes like benzene. The agitated man says an obvious prayer. Will his prayer keep the plane from plummeting? I make a decision that I don't have anything or anyone to pray to. I wonder if that means I am the only one who won't survive a crash. More Americans than ever believe in the Archdiocese version of Hell. Even Protestants. That's funny until translated into politics, into research for AIDS, into funds for starving people in those concentration camps we politely refer to as ghettos. There goes my brain again—

* * *

So I'm supposed to leave for a round-the-country car trip to do readings for Random House.* I must be crazy but I can't bring myself to cancel the trip. It's like some Disney pill where I'll magically regain all my energy—physical and mental—to make a driving trip like years ago when my body was preinfection. That life will stretch like a blank screen of sky on the horizon to be filled with all my desires, articulated or not. I still want to puke. I've been feeling this way all week I think from the penicillin. Yes, from the penicillin. Otherwise I have to think it's something new growing in size in order to kill me.

[No date]

I think I got kicked by a tiny mule in my sleep. Got that bone marrow biopsy. All I can remember is the sunlight. Lying on a doctor's table while she is pulling from trays all forms of equipment, rustlings of sanitized packing clink clunk of tools and a wave of late-afternoon sunlight streaming through the thin blinds across the walls, counters, and her moving white-clothed body. I tried to think what it was about sunlight. What I was always drawn to comment on to myself yet never have anything to say about it other than its presence or lack of presence.

I have a horrible streak of that discomfort sensation around my neck, the fear of touch, the anxious nausea of having the cloth of my T-shirt having contact with my skin. The doctor is going on about her business not turning around finally she asks me to turn over lower my underwear and she probes my lower back, my hip, and selects a spot. Invasive procedures scare the shit out of me, actually it's not so much fear as revulsion at the idea of marriage between body and machine and horror at it being me who all my life lived in fear of a rough death by exclusion, isolation, starvation, homelessness, untreated illness. Something about a steel tube

---

*David went on his cross-country book tour by car, though he was getting symptomatic at this time. Hoping for inspiration to write again, he planned to drive alone through the desert. At the last minute, he decided to go with a friend, Marion, with whom he had a complicated, sometimes charismatic relationship.

pushing into my flesh and further into my bone and clipping a piece of that bone. It's an issue of privacy in the worst sense. I have never in my life thought of my bone marrow except in the idea of giving it to others who need it. But that's been abstract, that was more about sadness and needing to fulfill someone's desperate needs, to break their physical isolation. Like my intestines are extremely private, so are my bones, the marrow inside them. I'm embarrassed at having someone accompany me in moments like this. My body feels like a third person in the room, my mind a second person, my friend a first person, the doctor absolutely necessary. I'm self-conscious for my body. I'm still in disbelief at my condition walking into these invasive tests like a man under a spell having horror but propelling my body forward despite it, a slight sense of maybe losing myself forever down a road that leads to endless illness and suffering and eventually a shutdown of my body as in death. Like in a time tunnel that telescopes and contracts life and civilization outside its transparent sides going on at an excruciatingly slow speed, slow in purpose, slow in awareness or ignorance.

It's done, not so painful but excessive in horror. She lays the little 1 2/3-inch length of extracted marrow onto a large glass slide. It's pinkish with blood and looks fibrous like the texture of gristle. It immediately looks like marrow even though I've never seen it before, its qualities are in magnification even though I'm two feet away and it's immediately identifiable as marrow. With a lot of effort she slices it in half with a scalpel, it will travel in two directions for different tests. Cutting it in two creates a sound against glass, a sound, a grittiness. So tiny but powerful. Next day I'm still in specific pain, manageable but still a thread of nausea and horror.

I'm thinking, I'm here. This is the chair, the bed, the shelf, the television, the lamp. I'm still here. Isolation is preferable even if I feel I'm dying of loneliness and of this thing in my blood. Being out helps for a moment but the whirl of fear and need and the pressure to decipher it all and not know what it is, causes me to want to go back into isolation— At least the bed won't disappear, the television won't die even though it is essentially death.

I've been depressed for years and tears since Peter died and Tom's diagnosis and my own diagnosis.* When I was younger I could frame out a sense of possibility or hope, abstract as it was, given my life felt like shit. I've lost that ability. Too much surrounds me in terms of fears, attempts to confront others and myself for clarity, to confront death or illness or loss of mobility or my brain rotting or shrinking, the recent loss of mobility in that I am too terrified to go long distances for fear of death or illness in unfamiliar environs. Knowing I've been depressed, realizing the extent recently makes it all more confusing because I don't know, I can't separate what in my fatigue and exhaustion and illness is from depression, what is from disease. One feeds on another until I want to scream.

When Peter talked for months about something feeling wrong, feeling like he was underwater, some acquaintances of his, one a shrink, said it was classic signs of a depressed immune system. She was stupid.

It's A.M. in Bakersfield. I think this is the town/tiny city where some cop got shot in an onion field and then they made a movie that made millions of dollars. San Francisco for a couple of days—odd thing to be in a city after Death Valley. Doing the reading [Outwrite panel] and its aftermath was heavy. I mean the people whom I spoke to and the heaviness of their private lives— One guy started to cry and said something of his lover home in bed ill and another guy had to cancel his trip to Europe to go the next day to get an operation on his eye for CMV retinitis. What a fucking horror. There were others, all of it made me sad around the end of the night.

One guy showed up that shocked me. In 1985 I came through San Francisco and tried to look up a guy who worked part-time at the desk of the YMCA I had lived in. He was long gone. He was a guy I was friends with along with a whole cast of eccentric characters at sleazy Embarcadero

---

*Peter Hujar was diagnosed in January 1987; Tom Rauffenbart tested positive for HIV in December 1987, and David followed a few months later.

hotels. We'd all meet at this coffee shop and talk all night. Richard was the most stable. Anyway, he showed up looking great and said he still had all my letters (I was twenty-one) and little notes and drawings I'd sent him back then. Then he was gone.

Amy was great. Something about her. When I first met her and subsequently I felt those old feelings of instant deep connection like you recognize someone you once knew a long time ago. But you really know nothing. So what is all this? She's beautiful and sexy and smart. Those words are stupid because it's all something much deeper than that. If she were a guy I'd maybe marry her. It's some emotional trust even though I don't know from where—

Another fight. I'm sick of this. Marion and me going through heavy times in Bakersfield. I arrive at a feeling that I want to cut off and go for a while by myself but then we're stuck in this town, this car, this hotel room, etc. We were driving all day. In the morning before we left San Francisco, she called Amy and asked her to join us for breakfast and for some reason I didn't say no when she asked me if this was all right. The night before at the reading and then the candlelight march for AIDS I felt happy to see Amy and when I went back to the hotel I wanted it to stop there, not see her again until next time, whenever that is. But in the A.M. I figured if Marion wants to see her there's a connection there and she deserves to. But then she started torturing me with the possibility of taking photos of Amy and me. I had been sitting at a restaurant in the Phoenix Hotel, dozens of people around the morning before, and she began taking pictures of me and I told her it made me uncomfortable. She didn't stop. It makes me crazy to have someone photograph me in public. Always has. I hate being photographed in general and the only rare times I have felt okay was when I was comfortable, when I felt a bond or trust between me and another person and we had privacy, sometimes in a group of people if those people were all friends or friendly.

So anyway Marion starts telling me she is going to photograph me and Amy at breakfast and I start getting uncomfortable and tell her she can't take pictures of me and a tension grows. She says I make her feel like a paparazzi. I tell her I don't like to be uncomfortable having my photo taken in a public place. She says she'll just photograph Amy. Fine, I say. I was tense all through breakfast, which read as having fun by Marion as she told me later. So I can mask my tension. I don't think so. I figure anyone can see my tension but Marion says she didn't. I was glad when breakfast was over. I just wanted to get out of San Francisco, maybe back to the desert just driving barren roads all the empty sky like a sponge or in worse times like an enormous mirror to tiny things and circuits like emotions.

So in San Francisco, I went to a porno movie house and jerked off. It felt kinda stupid and human. An Asian guy sat next to me, was putting his hands all over me. I was lost in the darkness of the seats. I felt a little weird. You know, having the virus and feeling like my body is filled with the virus and having a strange kid playing with my arms and chest and a straight porno on the screen whirring away in the dark and feeling like I'm sitting miles away watching myself in all this.

I told Marion afterwards, told her the intimate details of the physical stuff and all the complicated things going on in my mind as well. In the end the whole experience went from casual, where I thought, So what, to seeing it as vaguely interesting or that maybe it was good to have a sexual moment since it's rare that I do something sexual. It's been months since jerking off. Maybe twice in three months. Some switch fell off months ago maybe while I was feeling so sick. I couldn't give a shit about sex. It seemed stupid and boring, at times the idea of it, the complications of it made me think: nausea.

But in the course of telling her the story it all changed emotionally by degrees and by the end I was sad and feeling a little jittery. The kid wanted to suck my dick but I wouldn't let him. He kept trying in the most ridiculous ways but I kept refusing silently, just with hand gestures or by grabbing the back of his neck and pulling him away. He finally said, Why not? I said, It's not a good thing to do. It makes me nervous.

I couldn't talk about AIDS. I just wouldn't let him do it. He wrestled with my fingers, slapping my hand as if to knock it out of the way. There was something sweet and sad about it.

When I tell Marion intimate things like this experience I have sometimes weird feelings about speaking candidly about details but then I tell myself that she makes no judgment and why should I feel odd speaking about details of sexual contact? I push myself to open the book I guess to show trust or what I believe is a trust between us. I don't know what trust is if I try and look at it closely. I always look into a physical/mental communication expecting to see a physical shape as if trust were a physical shape and it is not. It's invisible and it is delicate and it balances like a thin wire suspended between two points.

We were driving in the evening in Bakersfield trying to find a place to eat. It's all industrial prairie where we were. Then suddenly suburbs and a small highway. She was talking about travel in Marrakech and getting picked up by two guys, French men. She was young and they all drank together. She was attracted to one of them and figured they'd fuck that evening. When she got to the part about the hotel room and smoking pot and then having sex with them she suddenly stopped and said, Oh I can't tell you that. It was a point of intimate detail, some memory of rawness and drunken high bawdiness I guess, and I said, Oh come on, you have to tell me. I tell you the details of my experiences. She said, No No No, laughing. I felt upset suddenly. Like a moment where something takes place and you suddenly have a view of how someone sees you and it's so far away from how you grew to believe they saw you. For me it was a shock. I felt something like emotional betrayal, like a laboratory specimen who'd been under examination in intimate detail by someone. Regret. I wished I could take back what I'd given because it was a constructed trust that I suddenly felt was based on a nonexistent foundation. Or that somehow the foundation was all my projection based on misinterpreted signs or gestures. I told her I would never again talk about intimate details of certain experiences if she couldn't tell me about hers. I felt emotional in this. Hurt. I wanted her to hear me. It was a flurry of emotions and it swept into the moving car.

It's moments like this that I wish I were a thousand miles into a remote place, unreachable and untouchable, devoid of humans, closing the walls around me to all people, speaking to the emptiness of the landscape or to the tiny workings of the world like bugs and animals and wind flowing and movements and shiftings of sand and sky. It drives me crazy not to be alone in these moments and for the rest of the evening it was that insufferable silence and weight: two people with two reactive versions of what events translate into. She said the fact I pushed her to speak of the details made her suddenly freeze and unable to remember or that she needed time or something. This was in the moment she'd been laughing and saying no to my prodding. Then she had a reaction to my being upset.

We went to this stupid steak house in the middle of a dead street and it was so hetero-inspired: crushed velvet walls with lumber, stained and burned, nailed all over the walls in fake western fashion, a handful of drunks at the tiny bar, and remote waitresses who could see we were outsiders. And a few tables of large families, moms and dads and kids. Everyone knew each other. And there we were in dead silence, like a fucking gloom cloud surrounding the table. If anyone wondered who we were or what our relationship was, it would have looked like two accidental strangers sitting at a table as if by all accounts of gestures and movements and sippings and chewing and casting our eyes about the ugly room that neither of us was visible to the other.

Those are moments I want to disappear, be in a car in the evening flooring the gas pedal, coasting into the unknown and nothingness of the desert or small cities, to be anonymous and unaccountable to anything or anyone. The only responsibilities are gas in the car, food in my belly, and movement to ease all that I carry. Let the vehicle, the sounds of night and trucks and the tiny movements of light distract me from my own humanity, my own body as long as I'm not sick, as long as I have freedom for my body, as long as I have my hand on the steering wheel, then I can drift and drift and even in extreme weariness I can prevent myself from stopping, driving into exhaustion, letting the mind chatter or die, whichever road it takes in the midst of all these thoughts. This is the problem with making plans that extend into the future with others. It's an almost futile gesture because it assumes a shape and structure in emptiness. It builds a psychic house that can elongate into what has never happened and to trust it is to be surprised by its arrival or to be darkened by its failure. At moments I wish to be alone but it's too complicated and I'm disgusted by the fact that I can't disappear and that all of this remains so constant.

Three junkies on TV followed by a cameraman as they work daily as thieves and live with women who are pregnant and whom one of them beats viciously on camera— The violent one eventually gets put away in jail for longer and longer periods of time because of violent activities inside jail. Fifty rules and he has broken at least half of them. I'm glad for his fucked-up wife. There's something sick about watching people disintegrate on evening television and yet it is compelling enough to be unable to stop or turn the channel or leave the room. It's like having an eyeball that hovers in space in the rooms of other people's lives, which are always fascinating even when it's mundane.

I also understand perfectly that it was a moment for Marion when she may have crossed a line emotionally and suddenly was self-conscious in the same ways I am in revealing intimate details of sexuality the point where I calm myself with the absurdity of the world and push on. She simply got hung up and I told her I'm not really interested in pushing her to go on and tell me what took place between these two guys and her body, I really wasn't. I don't have a need for those details but if I hear or witness them I simply add them to the construction of the world, to humanity itself and all its complications and forget it. For me it wasn't the information but the moment of what felt to me like trust broken. Not just that, but feeling another's gaze as being not what I believed it was. My emotional reaction was betrayal and regret, stupid as that may look at a later date. I felt like either I was a stranger or she was a stranger in that moment. It could be a child's thoughts, it could be. But it's there and I felt a door closing between us, not a door that covered all of our experiences but the complicated part of us that compelled me to open up and turn on a light to illuminate a tiny part of myself and my complicated movements.

I'm speaking of my sexuality in all its varied forms in the thousands of minute turnings of the brain and its body vehicle, the pathos, the sad lonely gestures between humans, strangers, in order to switch off the outside world. All my life I have almost never spoken of these moments, all my life I carried these deep in my belly. I never fucked people in a social community.

I always had sex with strangers outside that social community except for four relationships, half of them brief. I did this because of complex feelings of people who constantly verbalized and measured publicly others' sexual leanings. I told Marion that I hated the idea of people approaching me because they heard I fucked a certain way or that my dick was a certain size or any of that. I guess it relates to years as a hustler and wanting never to go back to that sensation of being meat or object unless it was a mutual desire.

Anyway, where am I? Sitting in a Days Inn in Bakersfield with oil pumps down the road swinging like enormous black insects ramming oil from the deep parts of the earth. She and I are at a stalemate. I asked her at dinner if we could let all this go and she said no. I explained to her where I was and she explained where she was. I told her that the sex information wasn't important to me, it was the moment that I described earlier. I felt it was all clear—uncomfortable but at least expressed. When she said she couldn't let it go I felt exhausted and a little angry that it was going to take over the evening, which it did, and as we lay in our separate beds I wanted to be alone for hours days months years, whatever. In the worst of it I thought how stupid that I break my isolation and yet I know my years of isolation were both painful as well as a time of need, that I learned something essential in that isolation but that it had a destructive quality to it and it made being in the world more difficult at times. So here we are. I couldn't bear to go to Death Valley with this stuff in the air. I would feel very angry to do that, to play a vacation routine and feel she could separate and do what she wanted while I felt like darkness. She has that ability. The only time I have that ability is if I separate and have endless time in front of me. I told her I couldn't go. That we should head back to New Mexico, stay in cheap hotels so that if the days were heavy, the costs would be low. To spend a bunch of money in a miserable environment would aggravate it all for me. I feel responsible because she has no car or anything and who knows how much money. But I refuse to be the chauffeur in a miserable voyage. I just can't do it. I need for myself to have some quiet days free of tension or at least as free of tension as is possible at this point. I have to go back to NYC and go into experimental drug treatments in Boston. I have to have blood taken every two days for a month and a half. It's gonna be a complicated season. Summer is hell.

When she was coming with me, all my thoughts were based in old memories of the exciting times, the intense communications that ran deep between us. Years ago we were almost inseparable. Others were jealous of us because there was a great sense of reality between two people that outlined something of the soul, previous travelers who recognize each other in the cloak of strangers. Two strangers who know each other intimately and instantly upon meeting. Maybe that's why it breaks so powerfully. But this time has been different. I can recognize what I loved in her in the past but something has changed. I look at her in odd moments and realize what a great human being she is, but I see her in the distance. Always. And I try to understand the sensation and keep thinking it has to do with my mortality, my slow death, my depressions in the last couple years. It feels like it keeps boiling down to my sense of mortality, the sense that no one else can touch something essential in me. Whatever she or others can touch in me, no matter how deep or rare, there is still a place, a form, an area below that that has grown in time and is untouchable. Their fingers are not long enough. No, that's stupid. Their perceptions and references could never grow long enough. She can't conceive of what I see or sense or carry other than that which everyone is capable of perceiving if they have the guts or energy. This is something different, special, unwanted on my part, undesired, hated at times, this view of my death, this slow separation from the physical disintegration.

I never feel sad when I see a dead skunk in the road the way I feel about other forms of life: birds cats dogs small mammals snakes lizards. Maybe it's because the stench of its death is so powerful it overwhelms me with the reality of its death. It stays with me for miles. So it marked the event of its death in such a way so that one cannot ignore its life. And the ending of that life. I need to think more about this.

I called the desk and told them we'd stay a second night. I told her I couldn't make a decision of what to do. Not with a half hour remaining before check-out. I'd told her this morning that I wouldn't go to Death Valley and pay the money for an expensive hotel room surrounded by isolation going through the motions of two of us traveling with heavy shit suspended in the air. It's something uncomfortable in me. I suspect she can detach enough to enjoy herself while I can't. I want to be removed, to locate something of a distraction, but to be in a motel with all the evidence of her presence and to have to move in a series of motions and constantly deny the heavy air for myself—I won't participate in that.

Later she said she would separate from me if it was what I decided and that I should sit with her and plan out the bus routes back to Albuquerque. It's all blank desert out there, buses may not ever go where she wants. I felt stuck. I don't have the energy to plan her trip, to plan the disintegration of this one. What is this? I just can't. I would feel angry to do this. I feel like I'm standing in the distance watching this accelerate and grow and implode and yet it seems stupid, what it's all based on. It feels like neither of us will move it to free us up. Like I said, I see it from a distance and it's sad and strange and it hurts, but I lay back on the strange arms of all this and think that, well, life hurts and life is sad and will all this when it's over provoke a radical thing inside me? Will it end something that never really got started?

When in the past we were together it was so strong. I feel it's me who's changed and not because I wanted to. Something essential has turned and I wasn't aware of it. It's revealing itself in a way that I can't explain, but I sense it in everything. It boils down to that thing, that form, that location that's grown inside of me in isolation and in the fields of time and aging and death, inside all the physical loss in the last couple of years, the last four years really, starting with Peter Hujar's death.

You know, it's funny, if I try to describe how someone has touched me so deeply, the process of language fails me. It's like I never examined it close enough to build words around it, around the taste and smell of communication, the blood of it in my heart.

I kept waiting for the switch to be thrown, the close-up recognition that she and I had resumed what we dropped two years ago. It never came.

I saw nothing but echoes of the past, but the distance was always present. It's seeing the familiar but consistently standing outside of it, never feeling that needed sensation of it enveloping you, surrounding you, becoming something you can lie down in without thought. I guess that got to me. It gave me a little spark of anxiety that I couldn't speak of. To speak of it would make it more real and I don't know what the results would have been. Maybe that's just my fear. Finding no reason for a state to exist. Wondering why certain motions are in play when the foundation has disappeared and nothing is in sight to suggest reason or therefore meaning.

I rode past the oil derricks and blank dusty fields of the town. Trucks and autos and mean-looking workers. Fires billowing inexplicably on the sides of houses and trailers and sometimes an entire backyard in smoky flames. From the outside looking in. Came back to the hotel room and she's gone. Her bags still here. This makes me depressed. I keep feeling that it's her decision to make if we split because I can't make that decision. I do know that I won't participate in the state that it's in now. I don't think things are bad enough to split but I refuse to go through formalities of a vacation in order to give her what she needs. I'd rather be alone and feeling dark as all hell than to be with someone in a way that makes me feel even lonelier. This morning I was incapable of making any decision in what happens to her and me.

This afternoon sucks. I'd told her before I left that if she chooses to split that she should check out the bus schedules and go her way. She later picked up the telephone book and that's when I left and went for a directionless drive. I won't sit in the room and listen to her make plans for the final moments of being together. Am I weird? I just don't like that pain. I still have two legs and a possibility of mobility. Remove myself from the probes of discomfort. It's probably just as fucked up either way but I can distract myself for moments at a time in the drive. A guy with no shirt picking up pipes and refuse in a field near the highway: no feeling in me really, just a spark of recognition in what used to produce desire. But it pulls me away from myself for a split second.

Sometime last night I felt like crying. It's been a long time. Today I'm getting lethargic and a strange distorted sadness. Her key in the door. I feel like leaving again but what would that do? Just extend this shit further than it deserves. So what's she going to say? What am I going to say? What do I feel? It's all too much. She, if she leaves, wants me to carry her luggage to New Mexico. I don't want to. I don't want the responsibility of having to reconnect with her after all this. Its ending would have to be final for me because otherwise the confusion hovers over all of my future. So what if it's nine more days? I want release in the strongest way if this disintegrates. She always said in the past, even recently to a friend of mine, that when a relationship needs to be broken off it should be done strongly, sometimes that's necessary so that you can look at it, at yourself.

So she says she has her period and I should come down to the pool and get her when I'm ready to go to the drugstore. It's too far to walk. This place is so desolate and industrial. I'd be surprised to find a drugstore. It's just feed barns, 7-Eleven stores, burger huts, and drinking lounges.

Tomorrow I am driving back to New Mexico if this continues. She says she doesn't want to go to a city and wait out the days. Too bad. I'm not going to be a chauffeur in this self-styled hell. Maybe that's my cruelty, maybe it's simply my need to finish this, get it over with and separate so there's a few days of my own silence, not two people's fucked-up silences. I realize all this—the air in the room, the vacancy of what she and I were attempting, the sullen darkness cast over everything—makes me suspicious. I carry memories of our past and feel if some of those things come alive in the form of her gestures I wouldn't be able to handle it. Maybe I'll explain what I'm talking about later. To revive it in words right now would be too far, too much for me. It would make the end of this concrete. I just need to be alone as soon as possible, that's what I feel.

As a form of life I can't believe how fucked up humans are. Or can be. What is this need to erase all evidence of other people when the conflict feels unresolvable? I did this all my life since my teen years, even against my desires or needs. If the emotional state felt destructive, I felt it was over, better to be over than to repeat it. I don't feel it's a healthy thing to do but at least in the finality of it my loneliness is concrete and in no one else's hands. I can't be touched any longer, and that settles into the general sense of existence I've carried. Way outside looking in. Way way outside. Waiting for all sounds to cease. All movements to come to an abrupt halt. The eyes to go blank with light or dark. To become a window, a form like glass that treads through walls and down streets into the horizon.

When I am sitting with her, even in easier times, I feel I am a stranger, not her, me, and she doesn't seem to notice. I keep thinking it's my mortality, but maybe not. Maybe it's that I've been isolated so long that something died in me in terms of my sense of direction or the sensitivity of my body in space, among others, I'm not sure.

She told me she made arrangements to go back to San Francisco by Greyhound, I guess. We drove to a mall to locate a drugstore where she could get what she needed. Then a bank so she could cash traveler's checks. I felt annoyed to have to spend this much time with her. Yeah, I'm a selfish guy in moments like this. She says she doesn't want to go to war with me. I understand what she means, but I don't think I'm going to war. I just feel like she successfully disassociates from the situation and can start conversations about something totally inane like the book she is reading, written by a friend of hers in Paris. I tell her, Look, this is too much for me. That book is meaningless to me in the context of this situation. It irritates me to have a conversation when this is going on.

   She can disassociate and I can't and each sound of her voice has left behind evidence of her presence, brings the cloud back down. Does this have something to do with how much I care or how angry I feel? Are they the same thing? It's extremely rare for me to write about something like this while it's current, no less when it's in the past. My distance physically allows me a chance to sift through it all and then lay it to rest. I don't know, I just can't go through the motions with her and not feel the pain of loss at her presence. When she said she was going to San Francisco, old feelings came back. There's always been the pattern that she goes to my friends when she and I have a split. I used to be paranoid about it, less so now. I guess what bothers me now is the same thing about the evidence of her presence among my friends. In San Francisco it's that I feel she'll contact Amy and she asked me for Philip's phone number. So why does that bother me? It does and then it doesn't, or else I refuse to let it bother me much. I guess it bugs me that all this can't help but make the public rounds. Everyone expected it would come to an end again like the previous two times. It almost didn't, but then the events of yesterday and my weariness at the idea of finishing this trip in tension and then having to go to Boston for treatments and all that shit in New York with the landlord's crew wanting to bust up my place to replace windows and hot water system— Fuck it, I can't take it.

She said for me not to worry about her saying things to my friends in San Francisco. I told her it wouldn't have any effect on me if she did. She said, Don't be insulting. I just can't care if she did say things to people; it just doesn't change who I am if they think I'm fucked up or if they think I'm okay. Maybe a little less alone in the world, but I'm alone any way you look at it, and gradually feeling less and less touched by people. Phil, who died a couple weeks back, used to say towards the end how much he hated healthy people, people without AIDS. I understood immediately what he meant. It's that no one can stop you from dying and they remind you of your own isolation in your dying, in the events of death.

If death from this disease were instantaneous like from a car crash or bullet it would make it all more bearable. I'm sitting in a restaurant and eating alone and writing and the world goes on around me. The Bakersfield world. For a moment I wanted to tell her, Don't go. On one level I'd rather finish the trip, on another level I'd rather be alone. I don't have a strong feeling of being able to retrieve enough of a connection to her to make the return trip have lovely meaning. Something has shut down, maybe out of exhaustion, maybe out of despair, maybe I need a catastrophe or explosion. This is not clear at all. I just want it somehow to stop. I don't want to expend so much on what seems essentially stupid. It's strange. It's not what we clashed about but the fact that our perceptions and views couldn't lead us past it in some way. I could let it all go but I can't sit in her silences and heaviness anymore. All yesterday evening was enough for me.

And it depressed me to feel that it would continue into Death Valley, and for me ruin what tiny moments of release I had with that place when we passed through it earlier. Or to witness her disassociation from the heaviness while it made me fall deeper than the inside of the earth. You probably wouldn't understand. She can't seem to. I'm stuck in what all this feels like. I know I'm a neurotic, but I feel fiercely protective of myself. I feel and have felt for years that I may as well be alone rather than go through things like this. I never traveled well with others except Tom because we could separate for long periods of the day and each enjoyed ourselves or didn't feel strange. With most others I always felt caught in their drift. I felt tension at the way I had to go in their directions when my own style was much more spontaneous and fragmented. I would drive others crazy if I insisted they follow me or adopt my style and yet I couldn't adopt theirs. Anyway, here I am and once again it all feels like major sadness, again like I can't ever fit. I can't be fluid and slide past all this. I feel deeply fucked up and simultaneously feel like this is who I am and what I need to insist on. I have to give myself room regardless what it looks like or is perceived by even the people I love or want to love. What a strange and complicated place to be. From the outside I doubt anyone can understand. Maybe that's not the point anyway. Maybe I need to reach a depth in which it all pours out. I have fragmentary thoughts of suicide, images pop into my head of driving my Hertz rental off this unbelievably high mountaintop road we passed on the way to San Francisco or else the chasms in New Mexico outside Taos. But I would need a guarantee that it would be a final act. When I think of suicide it relieves me, relieves the pressure. It's done that for me since I was a teenager. I went years at a time not thinking of these thoughts but they return now and then. The relief is momentary and I know it's momentary and therefore not an option that I'll take. Not at this point.

Yeah yeah blah blah. So we kinda resolved the situation. It's not completely resolved but at least the heavy shit has been pushed aside enough to joke with each other. That's what I wanted, and it was a roller-coaster ride for twenty-four hours. Sitting in the lobby with some suspicious white woman in her sixties, shooting looks at me over her newspaper, like I'm going to snatch her purse . . .

In anonymous sex it's the consciousness that his eyes carry and convey, the weight and beauty of that consciousness whether a projection on my part or a clear reading of it in his face, his eyes, the small gestures of his hands, rhythms of breathing. It's never so simple as a dick or a mouth. It's every bit as complicated as life and death was before society destroyed it.

ON PHIL'S BIRTHDAY/MEMORIAL

I can't live like a "normal" person. I can't fake that I am, or forget that I am dying. I am a stranger to others and to myself. I am a stranger and I can't pretend to be familiar. I am moving. I am moving on two legs or all fours. I am a stranger. I can't find what I'm looking for outside anymore. I can't find what I'm looking for out there. I guess I can only find it in here, in my head, in my solitude, in my distance, in my new persona as a stranger. I feel like I come from another world and can no longer speak the right language. I see the signs I make with my fingers and hands. The earth has a volume, hell has a volume. I'm a blank spot. I'm a smudge in the air. I feel like a window. I'm a broken window. All I feel today is sorrow. All I feel is loss. I'm a glass human disappearing in rain standing away from all of you waving my invisible arms and hands shouting my invisible words. I'm disappearing but not fast enough. I feel this blank spot, a great emptiness inside of me and for a while it made me nervous. Maybe because of my sense that I may never work again, never have reason or substance to work or paint or make photographs or make things that have meaning outside of myself. In that state what I make has meaning that circulates inside rather than outside, which defeats communication other than with myself. I move through landscapes or among people and all I see are echoes, echoes of what was familiar not too long ago, but the echoes are a skin of what was once an experience or a moment of living while now I can't feel the experience any longer. With Phil's death and maybe my own in front of me I am left with threads, threads of intellect, of emotion, of desire, of impulse, of survival, of need. I feel this sensation is no longer good or bad, it just exists and I can't give it words but I decided to let it live in me as long as it needs to, even for the rest of my life. It's where I am, it's my location at this time like an invisible map, invisible even to me but I embody or carry it and it is now my identity, it is my emptiness, it is my loss of reflection in the mirror. I talked to Steve and he says he feels the exact same thing and he doesn't know what it is either. I was once so filled with a desire to live and now that's changed and my only desire to live is my fear or reluctance to die. I'm not ready. What does that mean; there's no context for that statement. Everything has been reduced to echoes—all memory, all experiences, all motions of light and wind. When I stand in the street it's as if I am outside *time,* that fluid thing that expands or contracts. Everything I witness sets off echoes that look familiar but evaporate before I can physically touch them. All your faces, the faces of those who are not dying have become echoes, too. The movements of your lips have the echo or transparent quality of a film made fifty years ago and yet you are contemporary. At least you have an echo of contemporary about you. Who knows? Who knows? It's all abstract and my life is somewhere in the middle of it all.

In this sleep I was walking around near some large white piece of architecture that felt like a university or cavernous space. Picked up a telephone and dialed Phil's telephone number and someone picked it up after a ring or two. It was Phil even though he's been dead for two months. I was so amazed I was afraid to speak of his death as if it would make him disappear. I made small talk tentatively, just completely overwhelmed that he was alive. Suddenly we were before each other at a table in the white building. I asked him, How was it? meaning death. What was it like? He looked at me and seemed to be answering that it wasn't so bad. I could feel what he wanted to say but he seemed hesitant to speak of it other than shrugging his shoulders and looking more emotional suddenly. I think I reached over and touched him. The small distance between us was charged with emotion. I was trying to understand everything in the world at once. If he died and was now back physically and able to talk to me, then death was a process that was one of transition or travel. I was so re-

lieved to see him alive, or at least physical and communicating, I started
weeping and then so did he. We cried this short intense clear emotion. It
felt like what I think grace is.

I had to piss and went to an old bathroom, mostly metal stalls and
shadows like the subway station toilets of my childhood. You could sense
sex as soon as you walked in. I went into a stall and big sections of the di-
vider were peeled away to allow for sex. A young guy in his late teens or
early twenties was jerking off watching me. I jerked off and he bent and
leaned through the partition to blow me but I covered the head of my dick
and let him lick my balls instead. I reached through the hole to touch his
chest but he backed away to clean up. I was so happy to have seen Phil.
Woke up.

I've pretty much isolated myself from almost all the people I know, especially since the last two months when I was so fucking ill—constant nausea, head pains, unable to shit for weeks at a time feeling that my system is poisoning me and having bone biopsy, intestinal biopsy, and blood work and doing all them drugs that don't do shit for me. For a while I was injecting myself with interferon, now I'm on steroids. They made me feel a boost for a week or so but now I have trouble shitting again, fevers 101–102°, nausea all day, on some days head pains again. I'm sick of being sick and it aggravates me to speak to people who have a degree of normalcy in their lives. I hate it when someone calls and I tell them I am sick and they go off on this mundane bullshit about what they had for breakfast or what their kid is doing or whatever. That drives me insane. I can't tell if it's just their denial or their humanity. Humans obviously can never fathom what suffering feels like; there's a block in the brain that prevents it. Maybe we'd be so filled with horror we'd throw ourselves in front of automobiles. But it's all exhausting. I see that the relentlessness of my illness is boring for others, yet I'm the one who's fucking enduring this shit and at times I *have* to verbalize it despite other's fear of hearing it. So, that's why I isolate myself. I can't deal with another, But you look good. It's not affecting me too much in how I look, but it's hell in how I feel, the quality of my life sliding down to the point that I haven't worked on hardly anything for nine months.

I just hate people sometimes. I'm sick of feeling like a fucking empty Xerox version of my former self. Myself of last year is gone, is totally away in the past, floating like a rag in the wind. I'm blank, I'm a copy of my features. I look similar to a year ago but that sense of living, of fantasies, of hope, of purpose, of need, all of it's gone. I'm empty in regards to what used to touch me. I have no fantasies, even sex is a blank for me other than recognizing beautiful gestures or bodies: my kind of beauty. It's a bore to think about sex or try to jerk off, my body just doesn't give a shit. People, even when I explain some of this, tend to just yak away about their lives or say, Why don't you go away, take a trip, do something fun? . . . They don't know what they're talking about. There is no fun. Being sick in a hotel in the woods is worse than being sick in a familiar bed. I've lost the faint degree of hope I always mustered inside of drift or fantasies. None of it works anymore. So what, right? It's just what it is and nothing I say or do can touch it. Nothing anyone else says or does can touch it. I'm empty, other than of illness and dark thoughts. I want to die but I don't want to die. There's no answer right now.

This psychiatrist called me at the bidding of a friend. We talked for about forty minutes. He asked me about my sexual activities, my depression, my background a bit, and other things (health). I was candid. He wanted to know if I had been into S/M. I was surprised at the question. I told him of my few experiences and how I realized with low tolerance to pain I wasn't into it. Sometimes a slap on the butt in fucking was interesting, but the mechanics of pain were not what I was after. When Peter died I had two experiences, placing myself into the hands of a sadist I met in a movie house. My memories of it are complicated. Kind of makes me ill. It hurt a lot and emotionally it shook me up to the event of death in my face. Or something like that. Anyway I stopped after a couple of times and thought for a long time about what I wanted. I guess with the most important guy in my life dying, and I remember feeling I could never live by myself or go through this world without him (Peter), I guess I wanted to lose control as completely as possible. I mean this guy, this sadist, had me tied to the four corners of a bed and he sat on my chest and said, You are completely in my hands, in my control, right? Yeah, I said. I can do anything to you and you couldn't stop me. I nodded. Answer me, he said. Yes, I said. Okay, he said, untying parts of my body in order to lift my legs up to swipe at my butt a few times with a belt. It just hurt too much. Later when he left, I took a long hot bath in Epsom salts and wished I would die and leave everything/ everyone behind. I was tired.

Anyway, I'll see this psychic next week. Who knows, maybe I can release some of my state of mind and get some relief. Death is nothing more than relief. That's what informs my desire to die when I feel most strongly about suicide. I'll give this guy a handful of sessions and see where it goes. I feel interested to try but also somewhere in my head I wonder at whether another human can actually touch me deeply as I seem to need at this point in my life.

Except for phone logs and lists of things to do, this seems to be the last diary entry. In December 1991, David got sick and was hospitalized for one month. He was bedridden until July 22, 1992, when he died in his loft on Second Avenue and Twelfth Street.